PAUL GOUGH'S

The Healthy HABIT

Learn secrets to keep active, maintain independence and live free from painkillers

Essential reading for people aged 50+

by a leading UK physiotherapist

PAUL GOUGH'S

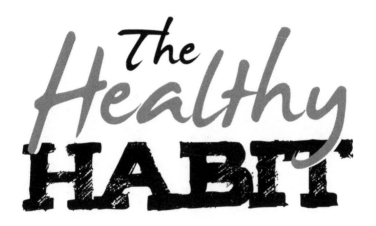

The **Healthy HABIT**

Learn secrets to keep active, maintain independence and live free from painkillers

Essential reading for people aged 50+

by a leading UK physiotherapist

MEREO
Cirencester

MEREO BOOKS

1A The Wool Market Dyer Street Cirencester Gloucestershire GL7 2PR
An imprint of Memoirs Publishing www.mereobooks.com

The Healthy Habit: 9781861514127

First published in Great Britain in 2015
by Mereo Books, an imprint of Memoirs Publishing

The address for Memoirs Publishing Group Limited can be found at
www.memoirspublishing.com

The Memoirs Publishing Group Ltd Reg. No. 7834348

The Memoirs Publishing Group supports both The Forest Stewardship Council® (FSC®) and the
PEFC® leading international forest-certification organisations. Our books carrying both the FSC
label and the PEFC® and are printed on FSC®-certified paper. FSC® is the only
forest-certification scheme supported by the leading environmental organisations including
Greenpeace. Our paper procurement policy can be found at
www.memoirspublishing.com/environment

Typeset in 11/17pt Franklin
by Wiltshire Associates Publisher Services Ltd. Printed and bound in Great Britain by
Printondemand-Worldwide, Peterborough PE2 6XD

Contents

■ ■ ■ ■ ■ ■ ■ ■ ■ ■ ■ ■ ■ ■

Chapter 1
Stealing healthy habits from the lifestyle rich

Chapter 2
Trying something new (especially at 50)

Chapter 3
Is retirement harmful to your health?

Chapter 4
Be kind to your knees - you'll miss them when they're gone!

Chapter 5
Exercising simply and safely, and feeling healthy doing it

Chapter 6
Healthy habits and daily rituals

Chapter 7
Unhealthy habits

Chapter 8
They laughed when I paid a private physio, but when they saw me walking again...

Chapter 9
Fatal health mistakes

Chapter 10
The death of good health habits

Bonus: your healthy resource library

Testimonials

■ ■ ■ ■ ■ ■ ■ ■ ■ ■ ■ ■ ■ ■ ■

"The success of this book is of no surprise to me - because what separates the great medical people from all the rest is the ability to communicate and motivate patients to take action - and Paul is up there with the very best and you'll soon see what I mean when you turn to the first page. What I particularly like about the book is that Paul manages to break down what appear to be complex and difficult lifestyle changes into "do-able" and easy to action bite sized adaptions that in the end, will make a positive difference.

You can read this book from cover to cover, or dip in and out as you need - either way, you will be able to make small positive changes that will help you feel and be better. For all those reasons, I heartily and healthily recommend The Healthy Habit to you and would any of my patients. This is a much needed book that a lot of people are going to benefit from". **Dr Chris Stevenson, Leading North East GP.**

"Chapter 2 gave me clarity on the back pain problem I'd been asking my doctor for an answer to for years – thank you." **Maureen Phelps, 71.**

"This book highlights Paul's unique, realistic and contagious perspective on the way that health care should be delivered - and because of that, Paul is someone the physiotherapy industry in the UK should be very proud of. I would encourage people to pay attention to The Healthy Habit because in all the years I've been in the medical field, I have to say that following through on the type of advice

given away inside, is what separates the people who actually win their health battles, from those who merely try for a while, and then fail."
Dr Mikael Peterson, Medical Practitioner, London.

"All I can say is thank you. I had been having a difficult time accepting that I could make changes to my lifestyle that would allow me to do something as simple as walk my dog three times per day - until I read chapter 4. The examples and stories in The Healthy Habit made what would typically be something I'm not sure I would enjoy reading - fun and interesting. Thanks for taking this very helpful information and making it enjoyable." **Doreen Smith, 61.**

"Many of the ideas I discovered in The Healthy Habit are quite different from what most people of my generation will have been told or currently believe - and that is what makes this book worth reading. When you pick up a health book these days, or even go to visit a doctor for advice, so often you hear about what to eat or what to take… there's none of that inside this book - just easy to take on board advice that if you follow, means you can make a big difference to your own health and future. Read the book and then pass it on to others." **Dave Walters, 59.**

"You will find more than nuggets in this book but a goldmine of information about the discipline of better health - the kind that makes you think you wish someone had taken the time to tell you years ago - because if they did, life might be much easier to enjoy. By the end of The Healthy Habit, you'll realise it's more about what you can do for your self rather than what any doctor can prescribe you that makes the difference. Read it." **Terry Johnson, 53.**

"As well as what to do, this book tells you what NOT to do and is a must-read for any person who values their ability to keep active too much to risk loosing it. What is delightfully surprising about this book is it's full of interesting and inspiring true stories - and little in the way medical fact – which makes it very easy for readers to enjoy and make sense of. As you go through this book you'll soon realise that Paul has a deep understanding of the health challenges his audience face and I'm sure that is what separates him from all the other physios and why so many people read what he says each week in his newspaper columns and are now buying this book." **Nick Loughlin, Sports Editor, The Northern Echo Newspaper (daily newspaper in North East England with a circulation of around 50,000).**

Acknowledgements

■■■■■■■■■■■■■■

To my son, Harry George Gough

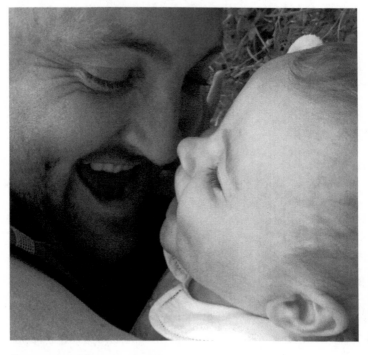

The happiest little boy I ever met. Everything that I do is done with you firmly in my mind - this book is included in that.

I love you.

Dad xxx

To my Granddad, George Stokle

The nicest, most honest and most humble man I ever met. I want everyone who ever reads my books to know about you and my only regret about writing it is that I can't send a copy to your house for you to read. I still miss you.

A special thank you

To George Reynolds, the man who showed incredible faith in me and gave me my first physio position at a professional football club aged just 22 - despite everyone else saying I was too young to do it.

George, I believe that most people can go on to achieve great things in their life if only someone would show them enough faith, or simply give them a chance – like what you did for me. I promise you, I am doing the same for my own employees now too - regardless of their age or what others say. Thank you.

About the author

∎∎∎∎∎∎∎∎∎∎∎∎∎

Paul Gough is an internationally known physiotherapist and founder of the North East's leading specialist private physiotherapy practice for people in their 40s, 50s, 60s, 70s, 80s and beyond, who want to keep mobile, active and free from painkillers.

You might know Paul as an expert columnist who writes weekly health articles for two of the North East's biggest daily newspapers, the *Northern Echo* and the *Hartlepool Mail*, and he is a regular speaker at health industry seminars in the UK and America, as well as a radio personality often heard on the BBC. Paul has been an expert guest on dozens of radio shows and is regularly interviewed in newspapers, magazines and trade journals all over the world, including *The Guardian*.

Paul's background included working extensively in the Premier League with a top professional football team. Since quitting his job in professional football in 2007 at the age of just 26, his physio practice has become the fastest growing in the UK and the biggest in the North East. It has been so successful that companies like BUPA and Asda, the Vela Group and Coast & Country retain his physio company's services to keep healthy their own staff and workforce. The Paul Gough Physio Rooms is now a large multi-physio multi-clinic speciality practice in Darlington, Durham, Guisborough and Hartlepool.

Thanks to his success in building an independent private physio business from scratch (from a spare room in his home), Paul has since become one of America's leading business coaches and top seminar speakers and has built a second business in the USA, where he is regularly hired by some of the USA's biggest physical therapy clinics to teach them his proven systems and strategies which offer patients highly specific solutions and more personalised customer care.

Foreword

■ ■ ■ ■ ■ ■ ■ ■ ■ ■ ■ ■ ■ ■

I first met Paul, reluctantly, in 2011. As my former tried and trusted long-term physio was retiring, I asked whom he would recommend in future. Without hesitation, he said "Paul Gough". Fine for him, he knew Paul Gough! It's just the way I am, but I'm a little reserved with people I don't know, so when I experienced horrendous back trouble and needed help, I was reluctant to seek Paul out, but I did need somebody.

Paul's immediate diagnosis was spot on and his expert, firm, hands-on treatment did the trick very effectively. His 'friendly puppy' approach (sorry, Paul!) was never threatening, nor invasive, and soon melted my reticence. His writing carries the same ebullient energy. His boundless enthusiasm for his profession and his infinite desire to share his knowledge with anyone who'll listen both surge through the pages of this book like a rip current. He has a great natural gift of communication and it's what he loves to do. And he has so much to communicate.

Not that everyone always wants to hear it! Much of Paul's vision is to spread a gospel of healthy habits as a preventative measure. After my back problem had eased, Paul told me to be particularly careful for five or six weeks to let it fully settle and get established in its recovery. I wasn't, and it happened again

- just as he said it would, if I didn't. I hadn't been reckless at all, just not extra careful. He was right – but kindly never quite said, "I told you so!"

Smokers don't like to be told it's bad for them and fat people don't like to be told a better diet would help. Similarly, sometimes older people don't like to be told how to live, how to exercise wisely, how to 'use it' properly so as not to 'lose it' in later years. Nobody likes to be preached at. Paul doesn't do it like that.

Just being TOLD doesn't do it for me; it can be oppressive, judgmental and accusatory. It doesn't provide the motivation to implement what you're being told. What can help enormously is when the person doing the telling actually comes alongside and shows an encouraging and supportive interest. If that person actually gives a damn themselves about whether you progress and succeed or not, THAT is a huge and effective motivation.

Paul tells it like it is, and tells it passionately. This book is very much in his natural idiom. Some of it you may not like, but – annoyingly – he's right! But helpfully, alongside being right, he does 'give a damn' about you … and that comes through. That's Paul. I can hear his voice in the words of this book, and people don't come any more genuine than Paul.

Bridget Boyle – a 69-year-old patient and partially reformed couch potato (as she puts it!)

Special bonus: gifts and goodies for health-conscious readers of this book

■■■■■■■■■■■■■■■

At the time of writing, more than 23,000 people from around the world receive regular and very practical health tips from me that are making it easier for them to make sense of the often very clouded world of enjoying great health and owning an active lifestyle when you are over 50 – via email.

If you'd like to join them all, just type this web address into Google: www.paulgoughphysio.com/gifts. Fill out the quick form on the screen and I'll also send you some other goodies and gifts too, including my 10 Day Healthy Meal Planner, loaded with recipes for ALL the family (Value £33) as well as my 7 Day, 7 Minute Stretching Routine Guide, which is perfect for ANY person aged 50 or over who wishes they were a bit more flexible and supple (Value £27). You'll be able to see them both instantly when you enter your name and email address at www.paulgoughphysio.com/gifts.

If you follow the simple instructions in both of the healthy resource manuals I'm going to give you, you will notice a positive difference to how healthy you look and feel. Go to www.paulgoughphysio.com/gifts to make sure you get them all (and I guarantee there will be more healthy gifts like this given out over the coming months and years when you join my email list).

Introduction

■■■■■■■■■■■■■■

This book is designed as a manual for *clarity*. It is written for everyone aged 50 and over who wants to challenge the prevailing assumptions of today's society and rather than viewing the second half of life as a time of progressive deterioration in mobility, independence and even "thinking", view the ageing process as a privilege often denied to many and a great opportunity for *increased* mental and physical activity.

The good news is that because of advancements in medical research and science, there's now the opportunity for more people than ever to live into their eighties, nineties, and beyond – with mobility, activity and independence maintained.

Thing is, so many people are <u>failing</u> to take that opportunity.

So why is that happening? Well, from my experience, I have observed three reasons why:

One - it's because at the first sign of pain, stiffness or restriction, too many people just accept it, think, "it's my age", or worse, mask it with painkillers. What's more, many people suffer from the disease of thinking *"it won't work for me"* – as if their problem is somehow different from everyone else's - and give up without a fight.

Two - because "bad" and "poor" advice is often sought from generalists, when a specialist opinion was needed. Worse, because of the ease of access to information freely available on the internet these days, more and more people are making the quick and easy, yet painful and costly, mistake of trying to turn themselves into experts – and paying the price in the long run.

Three - I believe that the biggest illness our society is currently suffering from is something called "instant gratification" – which, is basically, when people put off their long-term goals in exchange for instant pleasure.

An example of this: everyone knows that if you're overweight, more pressure is put on your knees and lower back. So one of the ways to ease knee pain, and therefore limit the suffering that comes from arthritis, is to simply lose weight! If you're a stone lighter, then your knees take less of a pounding every time you walk and knee pain will, inevitably, be significantly less. It might not go completely, but it will likely be a lot easier to live more independently with. Yet how many people are really willing to begin the process, and stick to it, of losing that excess weight which could make the difference they desire?

The problem is, losing weight takes time and requires discipline, and most people are simply unable to hold a picture in their mind's eye of how much happier they would be in the future if their life was less interrupted by chronic knee pain – the result of being less heavy.

And this is why people choose the route of "instant gratification" – preferring to mask that knee pain with painkillers – to which, by the way, a long-term dependency and addiction is likely to add even MORE weight (through fluid retention), and therefore increase knee pain instead.

So, if the person with chronic, painful and life-limiting

arthritis is unable to resist the instant pleasure of chocolate bars, biscuits and cakes – even knowing that doing so would take them closer to the outcome they desire – then what chance does that person have of being able to move into their eighties, nineties and even beyond with independence, mobility and activity intact?

This book is packed full with little-known health secrets - the type you're unlikely to be told even in a doctor's surgery. But just knowing them is not enough on its own. Ultimately, your chances of maintaining independence and mobility and living free from painkillers comes down to the decisions that YOU choose to make. It's true - your ability to make smart choices, overcome your own self-destructive behaviours and poor lifestyle choices will make the difference you're likely to be looking for.

Of course, it helps to have reliable and specialist information on the best ways to do that at hand - and that's just what this book is all about.

Over the next few decades, don't be surprised to see if real improvements in life expectancy (and quality of life) are less driven by medical advances and more by improved decision-making – such as reading books like this one.

An example of good decision-making for an overweight movie or TV lover might be to enjoy watching a film while walking on a treadmill. A long-term back pain sufferer? A 45-minutes-per-week Pilates class or a standing desk and less time sitting at work. A 55-year-old woman suffering with chronic knee pain? Changing the type of footwear she wears to shoes that might not look as nice, but do a better job of limiting the wear and tear process that is happening inside that painful knee.

Headaches and migraines? Some people suffer so badly that they feel like locking themselves in a dark cupboard all day long. The answer? Often it's as simple as changing pillows and limiting the length of reading time immediately before bed. Sounds simple? Health success often really is!

And as with most things health related, the simplest answers are usually the best. As you read through this book, you'll discover many of them.

Here's my first tip: have a pen and paper handy ready to jot them all down as you read them – that way you're more likely to take action. Best of all, most of what you'll learn you can apply to your life and start making a difference almost instantly.

Now, because I don't know you or your health background personally, I can't make any big or bold promises, but what I can confidently say is that by the end of this book you'll have clarity. You'll be in a position to be able to make a better, more educated and more informed decision about the future YOU.

It was my intention that this book would NOT be filled with complicated medical facts or terminology that will confuse more than it will impress – and I've stuck to it. What's more, there's no magic silver bullet, or never-revealed-before insider information that will change the state of your health and lifestyle overnight. Such a book isn't possible.

However, the pages that follow are packed full with simple ideas and little known, often overlooked suggestions to kick-start better health habits which, over time, and if applied faithfully, could very easily give you the health advantage you're looking for – even in your eighties and nineties.

If I may make a prediction. The problem you may encounter as you read through this book is this - many of the health habits I suggest may, at first, seem too easy and too simple, and therefore too good to be true. You'll be forgiven for thinking there's no point in adding them to *your* life because they won't have an impact upon your health, or assume they won't work for *you*. I assure you they can, and for most people who read this book, they probably will.

So, let's begin the book.

Chapter One

Stealing healthy habits from the lifestyle rich

■■■■■■■■■■■■■■

I'll start with a question from one of my patients/clients (aged 54). He asked me this common question:

Paul, I often find myself starting, and then stopping, just about every exercise kick I've ever been on. The worst thing is that I don't even realise I've stopped exercising (usually just going out for a nightly walk with my partner) until weeks later and then I find it difficult to get it going again. How do I find the motivation to keep active on a daily basis?

And here's the answer: you've got to know the reason why you're exercising in the first place. To find the motivation to keep healthy and active, ask yourself - what is it that you're actually hoping to AVOID by doing the exercise? Try thinking of it like this: is it to avoid always feeling stiff each day? Or is it to avoid infection, or lower the risk of heart and lung disease that are both more likely to happen to you if you don't keep active or do some form of exercise? Either way, you need to find something that motivates you enough to keep you from spending too much time on the couch, or in bed.

Now, your reasons for wanting to exercise daily may be something non-health-related, such as maintaining independence, preservation of self-determination or self-reliance, meaning you can still do things and go places for many more years to come (that's the driving force behind your exercise habits). And here's the important thing to write down: whatever your reason for wanting to keep active, it has to motivate you - maybe even scare you!

Think what life would be like if you didn't exercise by choice, as opposed to not exercising because you can't – for example because of some debilitating knee joint problem or chronic lower back pain. Whatever it is, paint a bleak enough picture of a life without exercise so that you don't succumb to the temptation of spending day after day sitting on a couch and in front of the TV. It has to motivate you enough to take action, however bad the weather is outside or however dark the nights are.

More: When I help people (usually in their 40s, 50s and 60s) who come to visit my private physio clinic, they often reference the ill health or inactivity of their own parents as something they hope they'll never have to go through themselves. I get the impression it worries most of them that it's not too long before it's going to be forced upon them too. And that's not what they want. Who does?

I worry about ill health in the future - it's something I hear regularly from people of a certain age, often the younger son or daughter (still in their 50s or 60s), who really doesn't want to live a restricted life like their mother or father, so they begin, sometimes for the first time, to really think about what they can do to avoid becoming so inactive or immobile.

And I'd be pretty confident that even the people who don't talk about losing independence must think about it from time to time. Do you? It's human nature to worry. And let's face it, we're very lucky that with health advancements and so much how-to type information on the topic of health freely available to us these days, we're in a much better position to stay active and healthy than our parents were.

I have a client in his 90s who comes to see me regularly. His name is Syd and he's from Hartlepool and I want you to know a little bit more about him so you can copy his best habits and way of thinking. Syd has no immediate family, so his independence and mobility has to be maintained by himself – currently with the help of a mobility scooter. He has no fall back and no one to do this or do that for him like so many others in their 90s. If he wants to go for a swim, he gets up and walks or waits for the bus to get himself there. It's the same with his weekly shopping or trips to the GP and physio. Swimming is a great daily habit which keeps his joints supple and muscles loose. It's great for his heart and lungs and above all, it maintains his independence and adds social interaction. He's always the first one in line too - standing in the queue waiting to get into the swimming lane at 7.30 every morning.

Now, I agree that life has to be kind to you in terms of illnesses and physical issues so that you can still be this active at 94. But, there's surely something in Syd's story, don't you think? You do? Good, then consider this: Syd didn't start doing this daily exercise when he got to 90! No, he has been swimming daily now for more than 35 years. You could say that's how he made it to 94 and is still so active. Something for you to think about, and believe me, whenever he comes in for physio or pops by to see me, I'm quizzing him relentlessly for clues or secret tips that he's used to keep himself so active and healthy for this long.

The hidden dangers of the path you walk on

Soon enough I'll come back to Syd and tell you some more stories. But now, I want to start to share with you some easy and very actionable health tips - ones you can begin to use right away after reading, tips which will help protect vital joints and help you to remain active and able to exercise for a lot longer.

OK, so a little-known secret about protecting vital joints such as your knees is this: the path you choose to walk or run on can have serious repercussions and make the painful process of arthritis happening inside joints inevitable. If you have a choice, uneven and gravelly surfaces should be avoided. That may appear to be a simple message, but here's why it's important for you to apply it: any surface that doesn't offer a flat, stable base will test your balance, stress your joints and your muscle strength and even your energy levels, all to a point where you could be doing more harm than good.

Now, in moderation, anything is usually fine. But the big problems come when you're choosing to walk the same path every night, week after week, month after month. Why? I'll tell you, it's because doing anything of the same kind repeatedly for too long just isn't good for your body. When it comes to being active (and walking or running) and keeping on the go for years longer, nothing trumps changing the surface you stroll on to give some muscles a rest, working some others at the same time. With that said, want to know what your best options are? OK, here you go: you'd be wise to mix it up a little and alternate between the beach, grassland and a nice flat tarmac surface and once in a while, hills or woodland is fine, too.

What not to wear on your feet

Next, let's talk about what you wear on your feet whilst doing it.

If you're more worried about looking good whilst you're on the move, then chances are your health account is going to suffer and deplete quickly. I've watched many women gasp in horror when I advise them to stop wearing high heels, which might look nice but aren't very healthy for vital joints, in favour of Velcro-style trainers bought from somewhere like Clarks or Marks and Spencers.

Now, most people know that the more cushion you have on your shoes, the less impact through your joints. That's obvious, right? But, what a lot of people don't know is this: there's also support and protection for joints to be found in the way you wear those shoes. Leave them loose, and vital joints move around too much, causing painful joint surfaces to rub together. But if you pull the laces or strapping tight enough, it can actually be a source of vital support.

It's true, the tighter your shoes are (but not so tight as to restrict blood supply), the less movement at your knee and ankle joints. And that means less rubbing and wear or tear of joint surfaces, therefore less damage in the joints in the long run. And that's why sandals or lose fitting type plimsolls should NEVER be worn when you're being active or exercising. Sure, they may look better, even feel better, because they're light and airy, but you're adding serious and unnecessary pressure to the joints that you need to see you through another 30-40 years of being active. Why risk it?

Next…

How to find a week's worth of spare time

Believe it or not, most people spend too much time in bed. And even more make the mistake of thinking that more time in bed equals more energy or alertness. It's a little-known fact that spending more than 7-8 hours in bed is unhealthy and a lack of knowledge on this subject is why most people lose what I call the 'bedroom battle'.

It's a battle that nearly always gets worse in winter when you might find it more difficult to get up and about as early as you might like each morning. And what should be the best part of the day can often be the most stressful. Some days might be different, but doesn't the day nearly always start off badly?

And that alarm clock that might be waking you up each day isn't helping. Here's why: the real problem with any alarm is that it's designed to frighten you into action. When was the last time you thought anything good when you heard a fire alarm, burglar alarm or ambulance screaming past you with an alarm sounding and blue lights flashing? Never, I hope.

So, an alarm clock really isn't the best way to begin

your day. Natural light lamps, soothing music, your favourite comedy show on the TV are surely better options. And what about the temptation to think you need that bit of, or a lot of, extra time in bed for fear that you'll be left feeling tired for the rest of the day? I know a lot of people think that way, but it's a myth - one you've been told by people who are just as keen to kid themselves as they are you that time spent asleep will mean more energy in the bank for later in the day.

And here's why most people lose the battle of the bed. It boils down to a simple formula: lack of vitamin D (sunlight) + extra time spent on the couch in the evening = feeling more lethargic. And that leads to the big mistake of thinking the answer to your energy problem is back in bed to get some more sleep. Rarely, unless there's an underlying medical condition, or extreme sleep deprivation, or you're a recently new mum, is this true. In fact, it could be your biggest mistake yet. The reality is that most people need less sleep. And more sleep hoping to feel less tired - well, that's a fallacy too. No matter how many times you try to arrive at it by sleeping longer, you'll never find the sustained extra energy you're looking for.

When it comes to sleep, less is definitely more. The average adult needs just 6-7 hours' sleep each night. If your current level is somewhere around 10, granted, any attempt to switch to 6-7 hours will leave you feeling groggy. But only at first. If you stuck at it for about 30 days, eventually it would become the norm and a healthy habit would be formed. And needing less sleep will become a habit that leaves you with way more energy.

That and with so much more time in your life. The real golden hours of any day happen between 5-8 am each morning. But how many people are still in bed or crashing around because they've slept in? Rising at that time each day could see you begin to exercise more, to plan and enjoy your day ahead and even clean the house in peace, if that's what you enjoy doing.

And if you do manage to make this a healthy habit, here's what waits for you: by climbing out of bed just ONE hour earlier each morning you will find spare time equivalent to one entire working week in your life, every month.

How to win the battle of the bedroom

I'll start with a nice little true story about someone who really is losing the bedroom battle. Here we go:

Could you do 6 .15 am?

It was a question I asked a potential client of mine who called up and asked for an emergency physio appointment with me because he was suffering with severe back pain. Believe it or not, the guy in this story said no to the appointment I offered. Why? Because he wouldn't be out of bed at that time of the day! Now, think about that for a moment: a gentleman in so much pain that he was unlikely to be able to sleep couldn't bring himself to get up and out of bed at a slightly earlier time than normal, despite the relief from back pain it would have given him for doing so.

It's so illogical that the only way I could think of to rationalise it was that most people are not lucky enough to ever be taught much about the real way to get the best from their sleeping habits. And to get the best out of sleep often means doing less of it than you think you need.

I find lots of people are confused by the issue of tiredness and the role their bed has to play in decreasing it, or, as they think, even solving it. No, rarely is more sleep the answer to increasing energy levels or feeling less lethargic.

By spending more time in bed (more than 8 hours is already about one too many) you will feel LESS alert and more sluggish. So, with that in mind, here are 5 tips to try that will help you get up and out earlier on a morning, leaving you feeling fresher and more alert for the whole day.

1) If you're going to bed anywhere around 10 ish, aim not to eat after 7 pm. This will help you sleep easily, as your digestive system will be able to switch off too. Take note: quality is more important than quantity of sleep.

2) When your alarm clock goes off, you've got to get up within minutes. Resist the temptation to hit the snooze button by leaving your alarm clock just out of reach so that you HAVE to get up.

3) Have a plan waiting for you so that you know what you're going to be doing as soon as you get up. Something like the first 20 minutes to get active, perhaps on a small trampoline or static exercise bike, 20 minutes to read a great book, and then perhaps the next 20 minutes to write and plan your day ahead (that little tip alone will make your day seem to last longer).

4) Set your alarm clock at the same time every day. That means Saturday AND Sunday. Understand that it's not what time you go to bed that decides how tired you will feel, or to be more accurate, the lethargy you will suffer. No, it's what time you get up. To find more time in your life and to feel way healthier, you must never change the time on your alarm clock.

5) Aim to be the fittest you can possibly be. It's no coincidence that most people when they get into a great exercise routine, often daily, will report both needing and wanting less sleep.

I agree, getting up early is going to be tough at first. And expect it to take about 60 days for any change in habit or routine to feel normal, even for the early morning grogginess to go. But the prize waiting for you for creating a good habit like this (and rising for just one hour earlier every morning) is the equivalent of discovering an entire week's worth of spare time in your life, every month. What could you achieve with that length of time?

Chapter Two

Trying something new

∎∎∎∎∎∎∎∎∎∎∎∎∎∎

Try something new. It's not as easy as it sounds, particularly if you're aged 50 or above. How come, you ask? Well, it's proven that when you reach the age of 40, the likelihood that you'll want to deviate from everything that you already know best (and already find comfortable), is hugely reduced.

Many people aged 50+ suffer from a lack of curiosity – and it's chemicals that flow (and surge) when you're in your 20s and early 30s that make you more open to trying new things. They are in much shorter supply when you move into your fifth and definitely sixth decade. What's sad about this is that many people get fear confused with a lack of curiosity, and it's causing them to miss out on a lot of things that might add value to their life and health too.

Here's a quick question: have you ever caught yourself

thinking, or even saying out loud, how fearless you were when you were in your 20s and 30s? Most older people will at some point in their lives acknowledge that they were much more adventurous when they were younger. And if that's happening to you – you're suffering from this too!

Being more fearful now that you're older isn't really what's going on… it's because you're less curious and so less likely to feel like trying something new.

Here's some real-life examples that affect many people I know: returning to the same holiday destination year on year, eating in the same restaurant each week and sticking to the same old fitness routines night after night. Why do they do it? It's because they tell themselves that they are happy doing it, when really it's because they feel safe, and doing something they know offers more chance of being happy (or so they think), and also makes them feel safe because it comes with no risk (that the meal or holiday won't disappoint). The thought of trying something new can make you feel *uneasy* at first and at the same time, make that couch and your favourite TV show, that chef's special in your favourite restaurant, that same beach you went to last year, or even that job you 'have' to get up for, seem more appealing than the pleasure each actually brings.

So what can you do to regain a bit of curiosity that might add something different and even MORE exciting to your day?

Let me offer a few suggestions…

Quality thinking time

Have you ever considered that driving to work (or anywhere you regularly go) a different way might add some sparkle to a mundane day - even if it takes longer to get there? Would getting up and setting off just a bit earlier be so bad if it meant you seeing some new sights or driving past a different set of people. It might make you a little more alert by the time you got to work! It also might make for a whole new conversation at work when you get there.

Ever since I can remember, driving to work a different way is something I've encouraged people to do – my staff included. My physio company has premises positioned all across the North East, so there are many ways and routes to get to wherever we all need to be and there are many scenic routes to places like Guisborough and Durham (if you haven't been, you would enjoy going to see both), and my home town of Hartlepool which is right on the coast, so it's a shame NOT to experiment with different ways to get there. Is there a better way to start a day than to see the sun come up over the sea? Or, if it's a bad weather day, watch as the waves smash into the rocks as you're driving past? (It gets pretty spectacular and dramatic at times when the North Sea wind blows in.) Admittedly some of these routes are shorter than others, but just doing a different one each day will offer something interesting and new to look at.

And here's something else I speak about at work to my staff: switching the radio off whilst you drive and doing the whole journey in complete silence, no matter how far you're travelling. When I first started doing this, it caused me some serious headaches. By the time the 30 minutes or so to whichever clinic I was driving to had passed, my head would be literally hurting from the tension caused by all the thinking I had to do. This happens because when you're not passively listening to the radio or yapping with a passenger, your brain actually has to do some thinking. And that's NOT something it likes to do. Really, it doesn't. Despite what you might think, our brains are actually very lazy and really don't like to do any of the thinking stuff at all. Has that surprised you? It surprises most people. It helps to understand this better when you realise that your brain is designed to get you from point A to point B in the quickest and safest possible way. That's it. And if it thinks you're not going the quickest way, the voice in your head will ask you why.

I find driving in complete silence quite relaxing too. Think about it, how many opportunities in your day do you get to listen to silence or the sounds of the outdoors? Very few, I bet! Also, I like to drive with the window open, even in winter, taking in all of the natural sounds of the outdoors and soaking in as much fresh air as I possibly can.

Admittedly, I'm a fresh air junkie. I sleep with the window open (even in winter) and the first thing I do if it's warm enough on a morning (or night after work) is to open the back doors in my home to let plenty of fresh air in. It helps to make me feel instantly free, and much healthier too.

Now, when you start asking your brain to figure out new routes to work, AND you're consciously thinking about something all the way to wherever it is you're going, your brain is not going to like it - at first. But your brain is not much different to a muscle in your leg which at first doesn't like it when you decide to go for a run or start some new type of exercise. The first few times you do it, your muscles aren't going to be able to do it for very long and they'll tire easy. But after a few goes, it's plain sailing - as long as you keep it up. Besides, whilst you're driving with no noise, it'll free up some valuable thinking time that you could use to start thinking about a few *different* things you might choose to do that could add value to your life.

It could be something as simple as going for a walk in a different TOWN (not just a different park), walking the same route but doing it a different way round (anti-clockwise), or perhaps something like taking up golf, even though you've never watched a game in your life and are doing it just because it looks fun and you might get to meet some nice people doing it. As an aside, taking up golf and giving it a try was just what my Mam has recently gone and done. She's 52, and I've never heard her mention golf in my life, so I was surprised to hear her tell me that she'd spent the morning at our local club taking up an offer of free taster lessons for ladies.

And why not? Fresh air, fitness, new friends, new skills, new frustrations and new success stories to share. Golf is just the medium to bring all of those good things to your life. It's a new set of circumstances, a new time to be somewhere, a new set of people to converse with and a new feeling for the rest of the day. I can't see any downsides, can you?

How to make it a healthy habit

OK, so maybe you're thinking about it and you're going to try something new. That's great! And if it's something that adds value to your life, you've next got to make it stick so that it becomes a healthy habit which will last. Now, I've heard variations on how long it takes to form a good habit, but I work on 21 days. That means you'd need to be working towards doing something 21 times continuously if you want that good habit to stick.

Answer me this: did you know that bad habits can't be stopped? No, they can only be replaced - by good ones. And I'm just thinking out loud here - one option for something new for you to try might be something like an organised Park Run. These events are popping up all across the UK on a Saturday morning (Google 'Park Run' for more info). It's a 5k run starting at 9 am each

Saturday morning and all (that means YOU, my avid reader), are encouraged to attend, including people who've never ever even considered running before. It's likely you will find more than one person who is your age, with your fitness ability, and who has your same outlook on life, at the start line of one of these park runs. They're great fun to be part of and also a great place to meet like-minded, curious people of DIFFERENT, but all ages.

But maybe your town hasn't got one? And that's great! Because it allows you to drive the scenic route to get to some other place close by and explore a different 5k route each week. These Park Runs are perfect if you're a keen runner, or wanting to pick it up, maybe just start up a new healthy habit, and perhaps are a bit fed up with jogging the same old route, week after week. Each run is an organised event, times placed on a website, starting at the same time every week (helps for the habit) and are nearly always packed full with people who turn up to just 'give it a go' and who are happy to try something new.

Last thing on this before we move on: I believe most people are able to go a long way to fixing the problems in their own life. The only problem is actually recognising the problem in the first place. So if you've hit a point in your life where you are constantly finding yourself *resisting* new things, no matter how safe or enjoyable they seem, it might help to tell yourself it's just the lack of a few curiosity chemicals that's holding you back and that life just might be a little more enjoyable if you tackle it with ACTION (probably healthier, too). And the easiest way to achieve all of that is to replace no with a simple maybe. Think you could do that?

A week without looking in the mirror

Whilst we're on the topic of trying something new, let's talk about creating something new.

First, a couple of quick questions: you know people go on diets all the time, right? As in, if you don't like your weight, you stop eating certain foods. Or, if your spending on credit cards was out of control, you'd cut up the credit cards, agreed? And if you needed a bit of quiet time, you'd maybe step outside and take a walk on your own, yes?

Now you could argue that these three are all diets in some form. And they are all good for either your mental or physical health. But what about your creative health? How much of that do we need? I once read an interesting book by a dancer and choreographer from New York City called *The Creative Habit*. The author suggests that most of us would do our creativity (and health) some good just by switching off from a few everyday things that lead to dullness and boredom.

And with enhancing your health and creativity in mind, here's my question to you: could you go a week without ANY of these?

- Mirrors - GASP! Think you could manage a week without looking into one? And I know what you're thinking: *What would my hair look like?* My answer… no one cares but you! And the reason why I include it? Simple. You'll be forced to stop looking at yourself and spend more time focusing on others.

- Clocks - Could you shield your eyes from one, just for a week? If you're engaged in what you're doing, time doesn't really matter. And if you're late for something*? So what!* Most people are too busy checking Facebook or just 'busy being busy' to notice anyway! And besides, if you are spending time looking at the clock all day, doesn't it tell you something isn't right with where you are in your life?

- Magazines - Could you do without knowing what's coming up on TV next week and actually wait for it to unfold in front of your eyes, learning whose dating who in the celebrity world or reading stories of other people's lives in the gossip columns? Just for one whole week?

- TV - How much of your thinking time is being taken up by focusing on who shot who or whose cheating on who in *Emmerdale, Coronation Street* or *EastEnders*?

- SPEAKING! Imagine a week without doing this! (and no cheating by sending text messages).

And there's a lot more. I'm sure you get the idea. There are a lot of distractions out there, and nearly all of them you and I can live without, at least for a little while. So, back to my question, could you go a week without any of these? I'd be interested to hear if YOU could, or have. Just use this email address to let me know: paul@paulgoughphysio.com is my personal email.

Try a new holiday destination

Let's imagine it's summertime for a few moments, and the school six-week holiday is in sight. It's the time of year when the British do one of the most illogical (even unhealthy) things possible, and that's go on holiday.

Why illogical and unhealthy? Well, after suffering through (and probably moaning about) an entire winter of dark, cold and damp nights, now that the sun has come out and the nights are long and light in Britain, most people start thinking about getting out of the country for a holiday. And by the way, something that I think most people in the UK take for granted is the fact that the UK is easily one of the lightest countries to be in anywhere in the world, during our summer months. That means if you're heading anywhere south of England, even Spain, the USA, Asia or France, you're going to be spending time in a country with less light than the one you left behind!

Sure, it might be a lot warmer, but when people think

of winter, the first thing they imagine is darkness. And as I've travelled around the world to various parts, something I've really come to appreciate about summertime in England - that we have an abundance of light to make use of and all you have to do is dress appropriately to enjoy it.

But going away and travelling to a NEW country is great - particularly if it's with family! And rightly so. Family holidays and travelling abroad mean different things to different people. For me, the beauty of travelling abroad to somewhere new has always been that it allows me to take a look at another culture and learn something from it. I'm not one of those people who likes to get 'away from it all'. I often wonder what people who say that sort of thing are wanting to get away from, and I can't help but think that anyone who thinks like that would be better off staying at home and putting right whatever it that they are running from – because it's guaranteed to still be there when the plane touches the ground in a week or two's time. And then it's a long 50 weeks or so until the next opportunity to get away from it all comes around. No, I much prefer to think of my travels as an *opportunity,* an *adventure* and chance to find some *freedom*, all rolled in to one.

Let me explain how I do that: I find adventure in seeing the world from another vantage point, and the sense of freedom in the absence of my everyday routine provides the excitement I crave whenever my days back home get a little mundane - which, no matter how hard you try, happens to all of us from time to time. And wherever I'm heading, as long as it's somewhere new, all the above nearly always applies. I love travelling to Europe because of the history and the architecture of the ancient buildings that I get to admire. And I like to get to Asia about every other year, just because I always leave with a better perspective on life – and feeling how lucky I am to have some simple things like running water and a roof that many westerners take for granted. I've travelled across Thailand, watched the sunset on Kuta beach (in Bali) at 6.15 every night, experienced the hustle and bustle of Hong Kong, admired the cleanliness of Singapore as well as the skyscrapers in Kuala Lumpur, even crawled through the chu chi tunnels of Vietnam's battlefields.

My two favourite places to spend time in Asia are Sri Lanka and India. I love the culture and the happy-go-lucky attitude of the Sri Lankan people, who are ALWAYS smiling and pleased to see you, and I love India for its humble, kind people, its vibrant cities and not to mention its great food. The only downside to a trip to Mumbai or Delhi is that once you've experienced their food at source, you'll never enjoy an English version again. I really do love to travel. And I have my Mam to thank for encouraging me to go and see places and helping to make travel a healthy habit in my life, from such an early age.

Before I move on, I couldn't do so without mentioning my favourite ever place to be, which is Orlando, Florida.

And more specifically – Disney World. When I was a child we would go often. My Mam loved the heat and the sun, but my Dad didn't. So we were never going to go on beach-type holidays every year. Orlando would allow my Mam to enjoy the sun, while my Dad could go to the great shopping malls and we played in the swimming pools. Then later in the day, we'd all go to the theme parks on an afternoon and have some fun. It's a tradition that I've kept with me to this day. I couldn't wait to take my little boy Harry to Disney World to see Mickey Mouse. He got there when he was just 4 months old, and I did it because I wanted to pass the Disney habit on to him too. I haven't got the time to wait until he's a bit older as I want those precious memories and experiences of him and me strolling the same paths that my parents and I did with me from the word go!

But family holidays aren't just about using a passport. Particularly not when the weather in England can be great and in summer you can be sure of some very long and light nights, particularly in the north. Doing something like camping and caravanning in the UK can provide just as much freedom and excitement as all the exotic destinations I've just mentioned above. But like anything else, you've got to be prepared to give it a go. And sure, if it's not something you've ever done before, you may find sleeping in the outdoors for a few nights a not very appealing thought.

Whenever I hear stories from other people of their childhoods spent on caravan sites or tenting with parents, it always makes me wish it was something we had done more of as a family when I was growing up. Now, don't get me wrong, my parents took me all over the world, which I'm grateful for, and that's where I got my travel bug from. But my parents weren't particularly outdoorsy people, so we didn't do much of the camping thing when I was a child. Aside from pitching a one-man tent in my garden a few times (I wanted a new one every time the latest Argos catalogue came out), and a one-off trip to a caravan at Haggerston Castle in Northumberland, I can't remember ever doing much of it. I think that was because the only trip we did take that time to Haggerston was marred by perhaps one of the few downsides I've ever come across with travel. That was the awful scenario of having to put up with a lumpy bed or a rock-hard pillow that someone else has provided for you, night after night. I've never met anyone who can enjoy their days knowing they face a horrid night in an uncomfortable bed.

My Dad was well and truly in that last bracket. He'd often complain about the pillows and mattresses causing some back and neckache, so much so that we never went back to any place where he wasn't sure of being very comfortable. Spending 7-8 hours sleeping on a pillow that's not as nice as your own is a common cause of neck stiffness, backaches and shoulder muscle tightness. I find it particularly bad in Asia, where they insist on big, thick and very hard pillows, in every hotel I've ever stayed in.

Is there a solution? Of course! I've recommended to many of my clients that they take their own pillows with them on holiday and I've done it myself. It's a smart move if you suffer constantly from neck and shoulder problems but still want to get out and pitch a tent or rent a caravan for the weekend.

Now, if you're thinking of spending some time in the great outdoors for the first time any time soon, be sure to consider the effect that a night or two sleeping on the grass is likely to have upon your back and neck, particularly if you already have a history of problems in either of those areas. If your neck or back is regularly stiff, it's important to start the day with some stretches or a brisk walk to loosen the joints to prevent a long-term problem (a good habit to get into regardless of where you sleep). Besides, it should be an easy thing to do if you're already in the beautiful countryside, as you won't need much motivation to get up and go for a nice walk when you're there.

Try getting active in a different place

Sometimes, that moment of inspiration you need to motivate yourself to get up and be more active will spring from a source you didn't see coming. And here's what I mean: A few times now I've travelled to the very windy city of Chicago, in America. I love being there, as it's one of the most fitness crazed cities I've ever been in.

What's great about Chicago is it's one of those places where you can't help but feel great. I'd go so far as to say it's the most active and fit city I've seen on my travels, anywhere in the world. Now, if you're not familiar with the geography of Chicago, it's a big city pitched right on Lake Michigan, which is huge, and because of that, it gets pretty windy – most days. But the lake comes in handy for the people who want to keep fit. There are designated swimming lanes in it with year-round life-guards (even in winter), running and cycle lanes, and one for walking too. As well as all that, you'll always see kids with their dads playing soccer or baseball (and basketball too), in the local parks. So, wherever you look, you're in the thick of people doing something that's good for their health. And that's great for you as a spectator! Why? Because just the sight of people being active and taking care of their health can very easily inspire you to want to take a bit better care of your own, too.

More: The last time I was there I was wondering around the Grant Park area one Saturday morning and witnessed all this I've just mentioned plus two fun runs, one for breast cancer and one for prostate cancer. I also witnessed and couldn't help but join in, an open-air yoga class with 2500+ people in the very same park (more on yoga later). When I was last in Chicago, I was speaking on stage at an industry seminar about health & fitness and I learned lots to further my career from the other speakers who got up to talk. But what I learned most while I was there was the importance of the *positive impact* people can have in helping other people in their attempts to keep active and healthy.

Here's what I mean: your children and grandchildren in particular will often need a bit of a push to get out and exercise – it's just human nature, particularly when they reach a certain age. And it's true that if they see you being active, then they'll likely want to do the same. On the flip side, if they see Mam or Dad sitting on the couch night after night, then they'll likely do the same as that, too.

Doing that is fine - it's just not great for your heart and lungs and it's not going to keep you very healthy, in the end. Your own habits are something to think about as you contemplate being more active and if you're looking for a kick start to be more active and healthy, try taking a trip to a random city where, everywhere you look, someone is doing what you wished you were able to do!

London is not so different from Chicago and it puts you in amongst good and healthy fitness habits. If you need any extra motivation to start being somewhat more active, remind yourself that doing so is not only great for your own health, but you'll likely be adding value, and maybe a few extra years, to the health of the people close to you, as they inevitably want to tag along. And that would be a nice thing to be responsible for, right?

OK, before I finish this section, let me tell you a story about something that BROKE when I was in Chicago. Just imagine this happening to you. If you didn't know, let me tell you that Chicago has two huge towers called the Hancock and Willis Towers. Both have those glass ledges you can step out on to where you can see the whole city beneath you from 1000 feet up. Believe it or not, whilst I was there once (though not while I was on it!) three people were smiling and having their picture taken with the city 1000ft or so below when the ledge cracked and shattered. As it started to crack, they all crawled off in a hurry, but the story made quite a fuss in the Windy City for the next few days and might have made a few people think twice before stepping out on one of those ledges in future. There is lots of video footage of it actually happening on YouTube, if you want to see it for yourself.

Why shopping can help keep you active

Every day I'm paid for adding value to people's lives by making improvements to their health, and I do it in the best way I currently know. Despite doing it at a top level for more than a decade, having studied extensively across the world and even been asked to write a book and publish my best health tips inside of it, some readers will remain completely resistant to the advice I give. So how come? Is it because they know more about how to improve their health than I do? Of course not! It's just because they feel that what I'm saying isn't appropriate or suitable for them – even though the advice is coming from someone who only has their best interests at heart, and only wants to see them be more active and healthy.

It's a fact of life - some people will still make up excuses and find reasons why they shouldn't take the advice or suggestions being handed on a plate, even if it's from an expert. And so it has be the work of resistance which affects us all, in many different walks of life. If I'm being honest, one of my big bugbears in life, and particularly when it happens in my physio practice, is when people make negative assumptions about something without asking any questions or seeking any clarity, before they assume it. I'm not sure if those people are sceptical, cynical or just ignorant, but either way, it's costing them good health and lots of enjoyment from life by not taking the advice of the people who really do know better.

Now, here's a little and very relevant story for you: A couple of years back when I was working as a physio in professional football I started telling my players they could shorten their recovery time, meaning they'd be ready for the next game sooner and therefore improve performance in the next match, simply by wearing specialist clothing immediately after they had played and trained. The reaction

I got from one or two was disbelief and a refusal to even explore the possibility that what I was saying might, just might, help. The majority remained sceptical and some even mocked the suggestion. Only one or two met my thoughts with enthusiasm and a desire to learn more.

Just a few years later, this new recovery clothing I had brought to the table is now used in a big way. And it appears that more and more top athletes in tennis, cricket, cycling, running, golf and football are relying upon it to not only improve their performance, but also to reduce the next-day aches and pains that happen to us all, particularly when you walk past the age of 40. And that's something that should be of interest to YOU. Because of the advancements that have been made producing this recovery style clothing for the top athletes, it's also had a positive impact on the type of clothing that is now easily available to regular people exercising on the streets and in gyms. You, perhaps? And yes, walking is included in that!

So, how does recovery clothing work, and how can it help you to keep more active and feel healthier? Well, the theory is that this clothing, because of the way it is designed and made, moves the blood around your system much more efficiently and removes the lactic acid that builds up during exercise more rapidly. This means your muscles are likely to feel less sore and stiff when you wake up the next morning. Lactic acid is that pain and burn sensation in your muscles that comes on towards the end of your exercise when you tire, and it's more noticeable the next day. Most people suffer from it. How badly they suffer depends on the cool-down exercises that they do (at the end) and on the clothing they choose to wear (or not).

Getting active in the outdoors

Did you know, the secret to <u>getting</u> fit is to steadily and progressively increase your exercise plan? And the secret to <u>staying</u> fit is to vary that exercise plan as much as possible. Yet the common mistake that people tend to make (which can lead very easily to injury), is to constantly pound the same path night after night when walking or running.

Here's an example of what I mean. Let's say you're in training for something like the Lyke Wake Walk, the Race For Life or the Great North Run, and you walk or jog on the same hard surfaces night after night, steadily increasing your distance each time you step outside. Do that and there's a good chance you will suffer from common injuries such as Achilles tendon problems or shin splints, even though you think you're doing your health some good by doing it. And by the way, you will be helping your heart and lungs, just not your joints or muscles.

Likewise, if you spend hour after hour on the saddle of

your bicycle, and you haven't prepared by doing the right lower back strengthening exercises, then you should expect to suffer back pain. Why? Because if your lower back isn't strong enough to support you in the seat as you pedal and climb a few hills from time to time (even leaning forwards as you to try make it easier for yourself to get up a steep bank or fight a strong gust of wind), then it will be stressed too much and eventually you'll pay the price with pain and/or stiffness. Even swimmers need to vary their training, otherwise shoulder aches and pains are inevitable. It's not possible to get into a swimming pool for an hour every day and use the same arm motion to propel you through the water without getting some kind of shoulder problem eventually. The swimming is fine, just change the stroke you do from one day to the next.

Anyhow. My BIG tip for this section is to <u>always</u> vary the type of exercise you do. As you've just noticed from the mention of how to avoid swimming injuries, it's possible to change an activity within an activity, so to speak, and it will help you keep active and healthy. Perhaps you could spend a little more time and effort putting together a plan that will work multiple muscle groups, improve balance, increase core muscle control (around your back), still improve cardio-vascular fitness (heart and lungs) and just as importantly, give vital joints a break. All you have to do is go along to a local gym and pay a personal trainer to set a programme up for you. Get this right and your chances of suffering from physical injury will reduce hugely. And that would be nice, right?

Now, this next tip is not for everyone. But stay with me as I describe it to you and you can decide for yourself if it's something you'd like to have a go at:

One RADICAL way to vary your exercise routine is to head to the great outdoors to test your strength, endurance and fitness in extreme but very stimulating conditions.

I'll explain how I do it and who I like to do it with. Outdoor Ambition is a company based in Darlington which I use to organise adventure days for my staff and clients. The company specialises in putting together packages for sports clubs, friends and families and even businesses to allow people to increase fitness whilst making the most of the scenic great outdoors. My team and I have done it many times now, each time a different adventure but always the same end result – heightened well-being. We've done things ranging from climbing Helvellyn in the Lakes, 'coasteering' at Marsden off the coast of South Shields and canoeing up (and back down) the River Tees at Yarm. On one recent trip I took my team, as well as some adventurous clients (all aged 45+), over to Middleton Teesdale, near Barnard Castle, for what was to be one of the most tiring, yet enjoyable, days I've experienced in years, as we took part in something called 'tubing'.

What's tubing, you might ask? Well, it involves physical

tasks such as swimming up the river against the rapids and bridge jumps from varying different heights, as well as walking, running and climbing up hills. And that was just in the morning session. Later that same day, having made it to the higher part of the river, we would spend the afternoon sitting in a rubber ring (ie the tube) and float all the way back down, with the flow of the river this time with us.

Now, maybe you're thinking that something this extreme is not for you? And if you are, that's great! Because now at least I've got you thinking about the possibility of it. And, if you did decide you quite fancy the idea of spending a day doing something active in the outdoors, but maybe not quite as adventurous as what I've just described, then I've done my job and achieved the goal of this book – which is to help you add one or two new healthy habits that will make a positive impact in your life.

The last thing to take note of is this: the key to the success of any outdoor adventure day is the varied nature of the activities involved. This allows people to gain fitness without even feeling as if they are exercising. And there lies the answer to the age-old problem of motivating people into staying healthy and active: how do you keep people exercising and active long enough so that it becomes a healthy habit? You won't need me to tell you it's really easy to sign up for a gym membership in January after a heavy Christmas period, but how many people are still going by March? Usually, not even half.

With this type of outdoor activity, where it's very difficult to turn back and you just have to keep going with everyone else, you'll be increasing aerobic fitness with the 6-7 hours of continuous walking as well as developing muscle strength from the repetitive bridge jumps. Swimming against the rapids and river currents is great for arm and leg strength, not forgetting healthy for your heart and lungs, too. Even sitting in the tubes on the way back down is hard work. Why? Because your lower back muscles (the core muscle group) will have to work hard to help you stay in it. In reality, this way of working these muscles is no different from sitting on one of those big blow-up exercise balls you will often see in the gym. The only difference is, you get to have much more fun, take in much more fresh air and enjoy the scenery as you float past – all at the same time. And you know what? It's estimated that this type of outdoor adventure activity will see you do more than three times the physical exertion you would do from spending two hours in a gym – and it's much more fun, because you can do it with friends, family and work colleagues too.

Stop 'exercising' – just find a way of being active

Let me start this section by telling you why I don't like encouraging people to exercise. It's because one of the problems that many people face when trying to get more healthy is that they think they have to do an exercise programme of some sort. In reality, that's not strictly true. Exercising can be tough – and even tougher to sustain – and if you're thinking exercise involves keeping fit, then the problem lies in the reality that you've got to keep at it. For some people, that's a big enough obstacle to even starting in the first place, and a reason why so many people look and feel unhealthy. They don't do much keeping fit, because they know they're unlikely to be able sustain it, so what's the point in starting?

Have you ever felt like that? I know many people have. And the answer? Well, all you have to do is to forget about keeping fit altogether. That's right, forget it! Because it's not the only way to feel healthier.

Instead, here's what I want you to do: just focus on *being active*. Same thing, you say? Not quite. It's a shift in the way you think and how you see the task at hand, and it will make it more likely that you'll sustain it for longer. All the health benefits you need, the ones that are going to keep joints supple and your heart and lungs in better shape, are often just the same as keeping active as they are in keeping fit. The only difference is that being active is easier to sustain. Besides, as with my outdoor adventure days with my staff, keeping active can be really fun, which means you're much more likely to maintain it.

Let me tell you something that most people don't know about why they can't maintain a *healthy level* of activity in their life. It's simply this: the way you feel about being active or exercising BEFORE you go and do it is never the same as when you're actually doing it, or when you've finished it. A big mistake is to wait until that moment when you feel a bit more like actually getting up and going to do something like take a walk, go for a jog or a bike ride, even go to the gym. Why is it a mistake? Simple - because as you'll have no doubt have noticed by now, that feeling which makes you want to get up and go rarely comes.

Now, a quick question to help you understand some more: Have you ever gone for a walk or run and wished you hadn't? Unless you tripped and fell, I doubt if the answer is yes! In fact, it's very unlikely that you will ever regret doing something that involves being active. In fact, because of the feel-good chemicals that get released naturally from being active for just 20 minutes or more, it's almost scientifically impossible to feel any other way than great.

To reinforce what I've just told you, ask yourself this: how many times have you sat on your couch and wished that you HAD gone for that brisk walk or nice jog, when the opportunity has gone and it's too late? A lot, I bet! The truth is this: you can only change the way you feel about being active and exercising once you're actually doing it. In essence, how you feel changes how you think. This, my health-conscious reader, is a better thought process to have when thinking about exercising or, as I prefer to say, keeping active. You cannot do it the other way round. It's a mistake in thinking that I see a lot of people continue to make.

The easiest way to change how you feel is to just MOVE. Do something - anything! Just get up and go, even though you think you don't feel like doing it. Why? Because you'll find it almost impossible to think any positive thoughts about being active while you're completely stationary. Your brain knows you're currently sitting still and doing nothing and it's too big a bridge too cross to get from a couch to a run or a long walk. You're giving it mixed signals. How can the decision-making part of your brain accept that you really want to suddenly get up and be active when you're stretched out on the couch motionless? It's never going to happen, and it's why so many people can't beat the urge to sit on the couch for long periods of time. They have no idea that it's even happening, or what to do to stop it. And it's a shame, because it's really easy. All you have to do is insert some bridges to get you up and moving around – bridges between sitting on the couch and going for a long walk. One of those bridges could simply be getting up and walking to the kitchen. When you do that, watch how much easier it suddenly is to make the decision about going for a walk or run, now that your legs are moving!

All of a sudden you decide that you now want to go and move your legs for a bit longer (and for further). Straight from the comfy couch to the streets for a long walk is a big bridge to cross - and it rarely happens. From the couch to walking around the house, to then taking a walk outside the house and going much further than you told yourself you would at the start, is a lot easier. In essence, you're playing tricks on your own brain to override it's resistance to exercise.

I appreciate that there's lots of critical (and cerebral) thinking going on here, and because people are rarely educated in making the small decisions like this which are critical to a healthier way of living, so many people fail in their attempts to keep active and healthy. Maybe the Governments and the powers that be should take note of this: it's one thing constantly telling everybody about the importance of keeping active and healthy, but it often doesn't work. Maybe it's about time they started educating people about HOW to achieve those benefits, and in turn, those people will be in a better position to help themselves.

Change the way you think to improve the way you feel

Here's a quick story that will help you if you're always struggling to find the motivation to go and do something different, but just never seem to see it through to the 'doing' stage. If that sort of thing is happening to you, as it does to many people, then consider inspiring yourself by looking for inspiring places to get active. In the North East and all across the UK, there's plenty of choice.

I told you a few pages back about my trips to the outdoors. Here's how I made use of the great outdoors by adapting an activity that many people do in their front room, or at a gym. Let me explain how. You've seen a rowing machine, right? Maybe you've been on one, or perhaps even ordered one from the catalogue to put in the front room and improve fitness (or lose some weight), whilst you watch TV.

As part of the series of outdoor adventure days I involve my staff and clients in, I once took my physio team and 12 clients canoeing. There were a couple of rowing boats involved too. We travelled six miles along the River Tees (and back of course), travelling from Yarm to Stockton's Tees Barrage, admiring some stunning sights and taking note of the wildlife as we rowed. The health benefits to me of having a healthy workforce are endless, and it might surprise you what can be achieved through a few hours doing an outdoor activity like rowing or canoeing.

Before I show you what they are, please don't make the assumption that I'm suggesting everyone reading this book is going to want to go and hire a canoe or a rowing boat and take to the nearest river, because I'm not. What I AM suggesting is that there is always another way to do something that makes keeping active and living healthy much more likely to become a habit in your life. By sharing stories with you from my own life, I'm just giving you some examples to help you think about how you might be able to adapt them to your own situation, to get the benefits you want that will make *the* difference.

As you read this book, there will be plenty of people who are sitting on a rowing machine, working out in a gym somewhere, or even exercising on one at home. I don't hold back saying this - doing so can be boring and difficult to sustain in the long term, but when you quit, it's your heart and lungs that will suffer. That's really why I bring these alternative ways of doing the same thing to your attention – to show you that there is nearly always another way of making sure you don't quit so easily.

In this example of me taking my staff to the outdoors to do the same kind of exercise people regularly do at home or in a gym, you can see how we were able to modify it and get the same health benefits PLUS get to see some new sights, hear different sounds, and all with the added bonus of some real human interaction (and fun) thrown in too.

Let's say you did decide to try rowing, either in the gym or on a river in the outdoors. Here's how your health would benefit from it becoming a habit:

● You'll reduce the risk of chronic neck and shoulder pain, as muscles in this area of your body will become stronger. Rowing stretches and strengthens all the muscles that can be easily hurt by having a poor sitting posture – a problem which applies to nearly everyone I know.

● You can reduce the likelihood of chronic back pain because you'll be strengthening your core muscles. You need your core muscles to help you out if you're spending a lot of time sitting at a desk or in any type of chair, or you've had episodes of on-off back pain in the past. Get your core muscles working properly and you'll reduce injury risk hugely.

● You'll burn <u>hundreds</u> of calories. My fuel band clocked over 700 calories burned from the six miles I rowed.

● You'll release lots of the feel-good chemicals known as endorphins. These are the natural drugs released during exercise which are responsible for the natural high you feel at the end.

If you like the sound of any of the benefits I've just mentioned but you don't much fancy rowing or canoeing on actual water, then head over to Amazon or Argos, or somewhere like that, and pick up a nice rowing machine that you can place on your front room floor to work out on while you watch TV! Doing *something* is certainly better than *nothing*. Unless you have a long history of having had a bad lower back, in which case you should seek specialist advice first, it's a nice way to exercise for 20 or so minutes each day. Enjoy!

Chapter Three

Is retirement harmful to your health?

■■■■■■■■■■■■■■

Let's talk about the dangers of being inactive. I may be wrong, but I think many people fail to prepare for what could be the single most inactive period of their life –retirement. If you're in your fifties, it's highly likely that you've thought about what to do in your retirement – many times over. Maybe even dreamed about it. But here's the problem: most people only ever consider the financial aspect of retirement. They fail to consider the other big, important aspect - what to do with the gaping time hole it creates.

So how do you go about filling the huge void that is created every day of every week, when your 9-5 working day is history? If you haven't yet considered that aspect of retirement, then let's do so now.

Start by considering how you feel about taking a break and going on holiday. Most people love the thought of having two whole weeks to do nothing, but then, about 10 days in, they start to think about getting back home and returning to their everyday routine. You see, doing nothing all day but lie on a beach isn't always as exciting as it first seems. Many people secretly get to a point well before the 14 days of their holiday are even up when they begin to realise they want to get home.

Your home routine is appealing simply because you don't have to think about what you're going to do to fill your day. More: it's happening because doing nothing other than sleeping, eating and drinking doesn't always make you feel as great as you thought it would. Somehow, the routine that you were so keen to get away from is the very thing you crave by the end.

What's more, have you ever noticed after your holiday how long it takes to switch your brain back on at work and be able to do things as easy and as effortlessly as you could pre-holiday? And your exercise habits are affected too. Think how long it takes to get going again with a simple fitness routine, or to pick up the after-work walks, with friends. Getting back into these good habits after a holiday often takes much longer than people think – if they think about it at all. It's not uncommon for three or four months of healthy exercise habits in the build-up to a family holiday to be lost completely when the return flight touches down at the airport.

So, what has this got to do with your retirement? Well, think about it - if 14 days is too long a time to do nothing, what will it be like with the 20 or more years of inactivity which is coming your way in retirement? How will you cope when you've got all that time on your hands and you're not sure how you're even going to begin to fill it? Sure, the monthly income may be taken care of, but have you thought about the amount of spare time you're going to need to fill?

There's not a day goes by when I'm not involved in a conversation about this topic with a client. Although retirement is a long way off for me, because I'm familiar with the health issues caused by inactivity during retirement, taking 'early retirement' is something I encourage people to think long and hard about. To be more precise, they may need to reconsider it.

Why? First of all, the health benefits of being active are endless. For some people, in fact I'd say the majority of people, being forced to get up and go to work is likely to be their *only* source of activity. And besides, it's a good thing to have some reason to get up on a morning and go and do something worthwhile. Now, of course, I'm not suggesting that at 67 you should be on a building site carrying bricks. But what I am hinting at is finding *something* to do, or a different place of work, or even a role within your current company that lets you have an excuse to get up on a morning and go and do something productive with your day.

The reason I say this is that most of the problems I see as a physio, such as back pain and knee pain, do NOT come as a result of being overly active, as people might think. More often than not they come on as a result of doing nothing. Muscles weaken and joints stiffen, leaving the person with the big problem of trying to figure out why, despite having done nothing, they're suffering and in pain!

Retirement offers a platform from which you can do a great many things that you've spent your working life wishing you could do, as and when you like. But I get the impression that in retirement many people just end up with a void. They have somehow been tricked, or tricked themselves, into thinking they're going to be doing all these wonderful things (and going to all these places) and health and happiness will follow. Worse, the reality for most people is it takes them years to figure out that this new, wonderful way of living in retirement is not actually happening.

I've heard it said many times by people who have retired that the hardest thing about being a retiree, and the one thing they really didn't see coming, is the difficulty of filling that void with something productive and worthwhile. It seems that if you're not careful, inactivity reigns supreme when you're retired. And, because this is a conversation I have a lot in my physio room, I've taken to reading countless studies on this topic of health and retirement. One of the most interesting suggests you're 40% less likely to suffer clinical depression, and 60% less likely to suffer a physical health condition such as back or knee pain, if you remain at work for a few years longer. It doesn't surprise me. This is because being active, even if that just means being generally 'on the go' all the time, as most people are when they're at work, helps keep your muscles and joints flexible - not to mention releasing those endorphins, the chemicals that make you feel good.

Now I accept that some people will disagree with what I'm suggesting. But I suspect that most of those people come from a position of not enjoying their work enough to want to consider staying on a little longer. That's a very different question to whether or not it's good for your health.

Let's look at a few examples: people like Sir Alex Ferguson, Sir Bobby Robson and even Sir Bruce Forsyth. Don't you think there's a reason that people like them chose to go to work in their 60s, 70s and 80s? You can't tell me it was for the money. You might say something like, it's OK for them, their jobs are a lot more interesting than mine. But the only real difference between their jobs and most people's is likely to be that they enjoyed doing them enough to want to stay on – and didn't have to follow the retirement rules and go at 65 whether they wanted to or not. Remember, they still have the same aching, painful joints as any other person in their 60s, 70s or 80s – and besides, when you saw them on TV or in the newspapers, didn't they always look well and healthy?

You see, from a physical point of view, the real problem with getting older is that every day you wake up, you're getting more and more stiff. You're losing the flexibility of vital muscles and joints, a process which started at the age of about 40, and as this happens, you're more and more likely to suffer from back, knee and shoulder problems. Keeping active, even by going out to do some kind of work, can help slow down this ageing process.

An example for you: I have a 94-year-old client (at the time of writing he's not my eldest – no, there's a lady whose 103 whose been coming to visit me since she was 94) who visits my physio clinic for what he calls TLC and a bit of an MOT. One of his healthy habits is swimming for an hour every morning and he is not only one of the fittest, but also one of the happiest people I'm lucky enough to know. Might be something in that, don't you think? Sure, swimming isn't work, but it's the concept of keeping active that I wanted to highlight and it takes a lot more discipline to get up and go swimming to please self, than it does to get to work – to be financially rewarded.

So, if you're in your 50s or 60s and starting to think about retirement, it's important not just to consider the financial implications of your departure from work but the options available to you to keep yourself as active as possible.

Here are a few suggestions you might wish to try, whatever your age, today.

It's always a great time to start something like a Pilates or yoga class, a daily swimming routine or join a walking, golf or bowls club – chances are there are some close by you. All these will help keep muscles and joints supple and most importantly, keep your mind active and sharp.

The blunt reality is that most people put good things like this off, thinking there'll be plenty of time to start when the retirement day finally arrives. But that's really not the best way to do it. Habits are rarely formed so quickly as to kick in the day retirement finally arrives. My tip is simply this: try to get into good, healthy habits as quickly as possible – starting today, in fact you've picked one up already by reading this book! In doing so, you're going to give yourself the best chance you can of being active, healthy and happy, not only in your 50s and 60s but deep into your retirement.

Has your job caused you problems?

If you are still at work, and plan to be for a few more years to come, let's consider the impact your current job is having upon your health. This section is important, because hidden inside every occupation there is a risk of injury or physical ill health. I want you to be aware of that, so you can avoid or limit the effect they may have on your ability to keep active and on the go for years to come.

What's interesting to note here is that most people go to work every day blissfully unaware that what they do and the way they do it is making it very likely that they will suffer from some kind of physical ill health. Let's point a few out and see if you can avoid them.

Plumbers, bricklayers, joiners and plasterers are all aware of the likelihood of injuries to their wrists, backs or knees. It comes with the territory and is obvious for all to see, as such tradesmen spend hours in awkward positions trying to fix things in your home, or on a building site. But what about the not so obviously 'harmful to health' occupations? What if your job is in admin and you sit at a desk all day, or maybe you're a hairdresser or dentist who spends hours stooping over their clients? These jobs come with their dangers too. What if you're a health care worker, a nurse or a teacher? You might be surprised to learn that such professionals are regular visitors to my physio clinic. And here's why: most people are aware of, or have been told about, the dangers of sitting in the wrong position for too long (ie slouching). I bet that if you've ever worked in a big office, you've had countless 'workstation assessments' carried out, or you've had it pointed out by your health and safety person that you should be sitting upright in your chair with all your body parts at 90 degrees!

But what most people don't realise is this: you're more likely to suffer problems with your lower back in particular if you spend time standing and then lean forward, or bend for a sustained period. And it doesn't have to be for very long. When a health care worker or nurse is leaning over a bed to attend to a sick patient, or a teacher leans forward to help his or her pupils, it's at that point that they are at the most risk of a lower back injury. See, your spine has to work nearly a third harder than in any other position when you lean forward. And if you're doing this every day, without being aware of it, you're almost certain to suffer with back pain at some point. It nearly always occurs in your 50s or 60s because of the compound effect of doing it so often for so long.

In a profession like teaching, particularly if you're educating the very young, you could have problems in the lower back area for many years because of a frequent need to stand and lean, coupled with long periods spent sitting at a desk marking books, and even sitting with pressure on your knees in a twisted position (as so many do). And by the way, sitting on your knees like this is VERY bad for you! The cumulative effect of doing it every day will often be the reason a teacher will suffer back pain or chronic knee problems somewhere in their 40s or 50s, meaning they will be less active in their 60s.

So, the moral of the story is this: whatever your profession, or however you make a living, if you're spending 8-10 hours a day doing the same thing, it pays to make sure you're aware of the health implications of doing it and the negative impact it might be having upon your health. More importantly, learn what you can be doing to avoid it (or change it) so that you can remain as active and as healthy as possible in your 50s, 60s and beyond. Of course, you will learn more about what you can do as you go through this book.

Where to find grand health opportunities

Ok, so let's talk about talking positive. I'm going to share with you the story of a turbulent flight I once took to Dallas, Texas, to speak at an industry seminar. I'm sharing it with you to highlight how easy it is to think negatively about certain things in life, when the reality is that there's a lot of good going on – if only you choose to see it that way. It's an unusual story of sorts and one some people would dread having to go through (feel free to skip to the next section).

So the flight across to the Texas wasn't great. One of those where you just needed to shut your eyes, think of something good and wait until the wheels of the plane softly make contact with the ground. But it wasn't all bad. Only the last 20 minutes or so as we came into land at Philadelphia Airport. From then on, the wind took over and at certain times it was as if you knew the plane's engines weren't in control any more, and the wind was.

It was the first time I'd ever felt we really were flying. When the captain gives you that pre-warning nod over the speaker system to buckle up, you know it's going to be a bit bumpy! And it was. But we landed and we were safe. And yet it was always one of those experiences where you secretly knew it was going be OK - you just feared what you might lose if it wasn't. Big difference. Massive difference.

And here's what I noticed: the preceding eight hours before the turbulence was smooth flying. Yet the conversation through customs and baggage reclaim in Philadelphia (where I was connecting to Texas) was all about the bad landing. Even though we had all made it, just about everyone focused on the small negative part of the journey. And so that got me thinking. I did some maths and calculated that about 96% of the flight was fine and enjoyable. Nice and easy to relax with a couple of drinks (and a book in hand) where you could enjoy the ride. Yet it was the 4% of the flight that wasn't ideal that everyone around me focused in on.

Moral of the story, and this section's big tip? Don't neglect all the good you've likely got going on in your life. For most of us, most of the time, our health is good enough to put to good use at places like the local park, woods or beach. Now is ALWAYS the time to make the most of each of them whilst you've got it good. For most of us our health is sound enough to enjoy a simple walk to or round all of these places.

I happen to think that there's a temptation for people to always think negatively about their health or situation. Sure, some people have got it bad - and I should know, I talk to people in pain and with ill health all day long. But most people's health is good enough to be put to better use and made more of (their choice of course!) I call it 'looking for grand health opportunities in your life to make the most of' - whilst you've got the chance to. A bit like the true story I just told you, it's often easier to focus in on the small proportion of bad things than look at the big opportunity for good things.

Sure, your health isn't always going to be great, nothing ever is, but I'd be pretty sure that most people have it a lot better than they realise - if only they'd pay a bit more attention to it.

How to make the whole 'it's your age' idea a thing of your past

Let's have some fun...

Every year at Halloween we hear stories of monsters, ghosts and goblins coming out to play. But one or two health monsters are lurking inside the bodies of men and women aged 40, 50 and 60, and these come out to play on a daily basis. More so, it seems, in the cold winter months. Their names: Stiffness and Tension. Both run wild in your joints and muscles, showing up when you try to lean forward (and struggle) or turn your neck (and can't) meaning you have to turn your whole body just to look over your shoulder. And although nobody wants either of them, very few people ever doing anything to prevent their impact, and not many will ever try to understand these 'monsters' or even face up to living with them.

And you know what? Some men and women even think that living with stiffness and tension is normal – accepting that just because they are a certain age, it must be an age thing, and they'll have to accept it. I've got some good news, because I'm going to explain how YOU can beat back both. But first, you've got to understand where both of these monsters come from.

The tension monster lurks when you're in bed and reading at night and surfaces in your neck and shoulders. The stiffness monster is lurking in your knees when you try to rise from the couch after watching TV for too long, and is in your lower back some mornings when you're trying to reach down and put your socks and shoes on – often failing. But the really strange thing is that some people will accept this ill health as if it's normal. And I've even seen some people who will happily put up with stiffness and tension in their body for 30 or 40 years. Sure, the battle with the 'stiffness monster' is a battle you can't win - and once you hit 50, this thing will never stop - but here's the thing, it wants *you* to stop!

What most people don't understand is that stopping

or even slowing down if you're feeling stiff is the last thing you should ever do. You can ward it off, you can even stop it dictating what you can and can't do. Despite what some people will tell you, stiffness and tension rarely go away with rest or inactivity, and neither goes away on its own. No, to win the stiffness battle, you're going to need to keep active and on the go. An important message for you to take into any winter season when the 'stiffness monster' comes out to haunt innocent knee, neck and back joints.

It's always worse in winter – my physio clinic will see a 20-30% rise in 'stiffness victims' over the winter months, each struggling to do the simple things like lean forward to pick up a TV remote, or get down and play with grandchildren (because they know they're not going to be able to get back up). I know there are men and women aged 50+ who, in the winter, fall into the trap of spending MORE time on the couch and LESS time in the swimming pool or walking around the park, stretching in a yoga studio or working on muscle tone in a Pilates class. And that's exactly where I'd recommend you be to help fend stiffness off.

Keeping active is the only way to fend off the unwanted effects of joint stiffness and muscle tension. Take action with the ideas mentioned above to keep active and you can ignore the gossip that says it's your age and you'll just have to accept it. When it comes to fending off joint stiffness, there definitely is a better way.

Who else isn't getting the message?

Let me ask you this question... how much of what I'm saying to you are you taking on board? Because I suspect a lot of what I've been writing about hasn't been absorbed, despite how important it is.

Let me explain what I mean. Failing to take good advice is nothing new. We are all guilty of it at some point or other. But what if that good advice is coming from someone like a GP, a caring nurse, a top consultant, a great physio or a respected chiropractor, each with a proven track record of helping to solve problems like the ones you've gone out of your way to ask about by visiting? How could anyone listen to the advice prescribed by a health professional and then not take action?

You'd think that because it's your health on the line, it wouldn't happen so much. Yet bizarrely, a failure of patients to take the advice of these sorts of health professionals is very familiar. I know for sure that many medical people spend their entire medical careers wondering how or why their patients didn't hear what they said, or didn't listen. But here's the problem for both patient and medical professionals (me included): in health care (but not limited to that field), there's a huge problem with communication. One look at the NHS complaints register and you'll see proof of this. It's partly because these days, people seem to want answers in record time.

Often time that through no fault of their own, health care professionals simply haven't got.

But the problem is not always the lack of time. It's often a failure of both parties to understand that however much time the 'patient–practitioner' conversation lasts, very little of the message is ever going to be taken in. You will remember as little as 7% of everything your GP, your physio or your nurse advises about your health. It's a proven fact. And anyone who's ever studied any form of communication will tell you that there are so many other influencing factors going on that the verbal message, the actual message of what the GP tells you to do next (for the good of your health), is usually lost in translation. Yet this sort of hard fact is lost on most health care professionals, because it's the kind of thing they skip over at university or in training schools. Sure, they touch on the importance of communication in general, but they never delve deep into the subject and leave with a true understanding of what exactly patients are picking up on (or not, as the case maybe).

It's not just in health care that this is happening. This 7% rule will apply everywhere you go today, in every conversation you have with any person you meet, work or non-work. It perhaps explains why so many wrong or mixed messages get passed on between friends and families. And if anything you do involves something as important as having to persuade someone to do something for the sake of their health, then it pays to know which is the most valuable 7% of the message and the 'cream' of the expertise you're offering them.

With that in mind, would you like an important 7% style health tip? You would? Good. I've already mentioned the positive benefits that regular swimming can add to your general health. What most people don't know about swimming is that there is also a very big downside. If you do too much of a certain type of it, you could end up with knees and hips that click, clunk and crack (AKA arthritis), more than you would like.

It's doing too much of the breaststroke that you need to be careful of. I know most ladies aged 50+ love to do it, but doing too much of this stroke isn't great for your knees or hips. To cut a long story short, your knees are not designed to rotate or turn the way you nearly always have to do when you're doing the breaststroke. But here's the thing... there is a modified version of the breaststroke that I'd like you to consider. If you like to swim and love to do the breaststroke, my tip to you would be this:

Take a float into the pool with you for a week or two and place it between your knees to keep them straight. Now just learn to kick your legs straight, without the usual rotation involved in a true breaststroke. After a while, you'll learn to do the 'breaststroke' without the negative impact of the rotation that goes through your knees and causes irritation of rough surfaces and adds to arthritis. I hope that tip helps!

Next – your knees.

Chapter Four

Be kind to your knees - you'll miss them when they're gone!

....

Quick question: are any irritating noises coming out of your knees yet? If not, give it time. Because, as you no doubt know, clicking, clunking and cracking are common, audible sounds that come as an inevitable consequence of growing older and they become more noticeable somewhere in the 40-50 age bracket. Chances are that if you're 50 or over, clicks and clunks might even be the first sound that you hear when you get out of bed in the morning. It happens to lots of people, and what's just as common is a grating noise which occurs when the surfaces of your knee joints rub together each time you bend your legs (or move between positions).

I could go on and on describing the different noises that come from ageing knee joints - it's so common that the question "Why does my knee click and crack?" is one of the most frequent I get asked. As it happens, is also one of the easiest to explain. So here goes: your knee's job is to cushion and absorb the shock it receives from the pounding, twisting and impact of hard surfaces every time your foot lands when you walk. Your knee takes a pounding from the hard surfaces you walk on, regardless of what else you do. Add this to the pounding your knees take as a direct result of playing a game of five-a-side football after work in a sports hall, running along the beach, playing bowls, golf, or just taking a long walk around the park or in the hills or woods with friends on a weekend. The upshot of all this is that, over time, this cartilage wears thin (or disappears completely), exposing nerves and causing pain but also leaving uneven surfaces that can collide – and because these bones in your knee joint are very tough and hard (as you might well expect), inevitably they cause a distinct noise when they rub against each other as you move your leg in and out of different positions. And that's it, nothing more to it. The phenomenon of knee joint noises explained in one paragraph!

What's interesting is that the presence of the noises doesn't always mean you'll get knee pain - not at first anyway. But it's often the first sign that trouble in the form of pain, stiffness and swelling is on the way and you're not too many years away from it. If you like, it's a warning sign to act fast and do something before things turn for the worse.

So what do you do about it?

Of course, you have the option of doing nothing about it or even trying one of those Neoprene knee supports, which might help (but only for a short while), or you might opt to go and see a good physio for some solid advice! I suggest this because knees have a habit of getting more painful as you move through your 50s and 60s, and you will benefit from something to slow that down – which could be a simple case of exercises to strengthen the right muscles to help protect and support your knee – done once or twice per day. Would that be so bad if it meant less painful knees?

To avoid, or get relief from, knee pain that happens because of a gradual wear and tear process (as I've just described to you), you need to be doing the right type of exercises, done in the right way, at the right time. You must be doing routines that specifically strengthen your muscles and add something called control. Without control in your knee muscles, the degeneration in your knee accelerates faster than a high speed train pulling away from the station.

Next, here's a word of warning. I hear a lot of people talking about their painful knees in conversations with friends. Because everyone thinks they have the answers to issues like this, people are unfortunately giving each other often bad and even dangerous advice, which is usually more confusing than it needs to be and often diabetes the importance of the message that something needs to be done – like physio.

Because there's a lot of confusion around it, I want you to know about this medical fact: there's a big difference between *exercising* and *doing exercises* (note: I define exercising as doing something like walking for 20 minutes per day, and exercises being a steady and controlled sequence of movements designed to strengthen or make flexible a specific muscle group).

One of the big mistakes I see GPs make is telling people looking for a solution to knee pain to just 'go and do some exercise', as if more exercise will make the pain go away. But, as you're about to discover, more exercise is rarely the right answer. Not when it is already painful, anyway.

You see, the BIG mistake currently being made out there in society when it comes to healthy living is to think that when knee pain gets really bad, doing exercise - such as running and even more walking - will help make your knee stronger and therefore less painful. It won't. In fact, exercise will often make a swollen, painful knee even worse. The only thing you should ever consider doing is to stop exercising completely for a short period and instead, strengthen the muscles that are designed to protect and support the knee by doing specific exercises prescribed by a specialist physio.

In case you are wondering, the muscles you should be strengthening include your thigh, hamstring and lower back muscles and it pays to have your feet looked at - just to make sure they're in the right position before you exercise too. That way, all bases are covered and your knee has enough natural support from above and below to let you do the type of activity you love doing, free from relying upon painkillers. Don't worry – I'm not talking about doing exercises that involve any heavy lifting of weights or sitting on machines (the latter I never advise), or anything like that. No. It's possible to strengthen your knee muscles sufficiently just by using something as easy to get hold of as a resistance band. What's one of those, you might ask? Well, it's a large elastic band that has different levels of strength (often distinguished by colour) and all you do is strap it or tie it to something heavy or firm like a couch leg, and continuously work your knee muscles against the resistance. You could even do a few simple exercises on the bottom of the stairs in your own home, or on a step.

Next, let's talk about...

The dangers of wearing summer sandals

Let's presume it's the start of summer and we're in May (which is national walking month), one of the most perfect times of the year to get out and enjoy the fresh air and the sights of your town. Now, on the face of it, walking appears to be a really safe way to keep fit and active and you'd be forgiven for thinking you're being kind to your knees by doing it regularly. But, there are a few things I'd like you to know about walking to make sure your walk is as enjoyable, as healthy and as comfortable as possible.

So here goes: how strong and flexible your lower back is will affect how painful your knees become if you're a regular walker. Also important is the surface you walk or run on, such as a hard or uneven surface, or a soft piece of grassland. And the one most people don't know about… what you choose to wear on your feet. So let's talk about the latter - and make sure you know everything you need to know about it to protect yourself as best you can.

OK, if you enjoy a gentle evening stroll along the sea front, or around the local park whilst chatting with a friend, then a simple pair of cushioned trainers will do. But, seriously, be careful with your choice as some of the fashionable plimsoll-style trainers offer very little support for your ankles and feet and will mean that your knee joint is likely to be moving around a little too much. If that happens, your knee bones will rub together, causing the wear and tear to increase. The problem is this: you'll never know it's happening, at least not until you see some swelling or feel heat coming from your knee. I assure you, your knee is under much added stress if your footwear isn't protecting it by absorbing some shock from the pavement and keeping it in a steady position.

A similar thing can happen if you wear flip-flops or sandals. This is a particular problem for ladies in the summer months who choose to swap their high heels for lighter sandals. Don't be surprised if after a two-week holiday when you've likely been wearing flat sandals all day, you suddenly develop a pain in and around the back of your ankle. If you do, it's a good sign that you've irritated your Achilles tendon – which can be a long-term problem that many ladies suffer from daily.

Walking along the beach or around the park is one thing, but if you're a bit more adventurous and like to walk in the hills or woods, or, you're a serious weekend walker and part of a group who do it for more than just fun, then your footwear choice has to be much more sturdy.

With that in mind, here's a nice little story for you. In March 2013 I took a walk up a mountain called Toubkal, in Morocco. At 4167 meters above sea level it's the highest mountain in North Africa and to conquer it I had no option but to choose comfort and safety over style and opt for proper mountain climbing boots. And you should too - even if you're not climbing mountains in North Africa, but are just regularly walking on a hilly or gravelly surface, you should make sure you're wearing the right walking boots.

Now, have you got a pen handy? Because I want you to make a note of this next tip that I've got for you, which might save you some frustration and some money. If you're ever purchasing a pair of walking shoes, the best time to try them on in the shop is late morning or midafternoon. Why? Because your feet swell up during the day and if you go and get fitted for shoes first thing in the morning, you might not get an accurate fit and end up buying a pair that seemed to fit perfectly in the shop, but are actually just a bit too tight when you put them on. And that's not good for comfort or blood circulation to your ankle joint.

We're nearly finished this section, but before we do, one final thing to note on the topic of walking: if you're already suffering from something like a bad or stiff lower back, or have arthritic knees, it's best to avoid hilly and uneven surfaces completely. For all of the good reasons I've already written about, walking on these surfaces makes it more likely that you'll have a more swollen knee, or an even stiffer lower back due to the extra pressure, stress and demands placed on your body.

To sum up: walking on flat, even surfaces is much healthier for your joints and will likely limit any problems enough to allow you to enjoy your walking for years to come.

Why knees get more painful in winter

Now let's skip from summer to winter. We're leaving the warm weather behind and moving into the cold, dark, damp months of winter. If you're in your late 50s or 60s, there's a good chance you've already experienced something strange happening to your joints when the temperature begins to drop. They suddenly get that bit more annoying, nagging and painful, on a daily basis. If you're struggling to put your finger on why it happens every year at the same time, I can assure you you're not the only one it's happening to. The sensation that knee joints appear to become more stiff, ache more, clunk more and even swell more when the temperature drops is one that many men and women aged 50+ can hold their hand up to having suffered from.

There are many reasons why your joints appear to be more problematic come wintertime. Two villains in the story are the low temperature, which naturally restricts your circulation, and the fact that you're much less likely to be active in winter, further restricting the blood supply. Yet keeping joints mobile by being active is the equivalent of spraying WD40 on the stiff and rusty joints of an old bike or car – it's essential oil that makes the ride much easier and smoother.

And here's the thing that many people in their 50s and 60s fail to grasp: the long winter months and a sustained period of inactivity can be the root cause of what I call 'all of a sudden' lifelong knee pains. You see, if your muscles get a long rest in winter, there's a chance they'll waste away to the point where they will not be able to support your knees as they once could when you start up again in the spring, when you feel more like being active. And without the support of the muscles, knees are much more likely to end up arthritic.

Here's what goes on: after a long winter of inactivity and hibernation, the temptation is to automatically begin to exercise again when the good weather and light nights come around. But your muscles may not be strong enough to suddenly start exercising again safely after so much rest. Not if you've shut these muscles down for six whole months!

The harsh reality for many knee pain victims is that most of their problems will be added to by a long winter break from activity. First you experience a lull in your exercise and then you think it's OK to go back to doing all the things you did before the break. So, with that in mind, here's a big tip to help you avoid making this mistake: seize any and every opportunity you have during winter to get active and keep joints mobile and vital muscles strong. If you're lucky, you'll never get to know what life with dodgy knees might have been like if you hadn't.

What not to wear, and why it makes knee pain worse

'Early retirement' - it's a phrase that brings nice thoughts of time spent choosing activities that suit you – early morning works with no time limit, sunny rounds of golf as and when, playing with grandchildren in a park, or just more time attending to the garden. Whatever it is, when you become a retiree, you're going to have a lot more time to do it. Now, as we discussed in an earlier section, retiring from a nine to five job has its pitfalls, and most people want to retire from their careers a lot earlier than they actually can. But what about retiring early from exercise or sport because of ill health? Some people, despite the advice they get from the experts, just can't seem to do it.

I've even seen at first hand how some people will refuse to listen to solid medical advice and are always tempted to give it 'one more go' at playing the sport that they love, or doing the exercise which they enjoy, despite what the experts advise them to do. Wearing something like a neoprene support is usually the first thing any person aged 50 or over will try - just to find some way of limiting the impact of whatever injury or problem they have with their knee in order to go on exercising for a few more years.

Which is fine. After all, we're just here to advise! But, the reality is, these supports are not healthy - not in the long run anyway. Why? Because whenever you wear something like a knee or back support, all the muscles that are being supported are slowly but surely wasting away to nothing. Every time you pull on a knee or back support you're giving your muscles a rest – which is fine for a few days. But, if and when that neoprene support becomes a forced habit, and you feel as though you can't go anywhere unless you're wearing it, then you're in trouble.

Here's why. In the first two or three weeks of wearing

a support, sure, you will feel a noticeable and very positive difference as a result of doing so. The problem is that for those three weeks the muscles in your knee (or wherever you are wearing it) have had a rest. So you have been tricked into thinking your body is getting better because of the absence of pain or swelling. But that's only happened because of the knee support. It will initially do its job and support your knee, yet in reality, your body is getting weaker every time you do wear it, and that's happening because the muscles are not being used as they were designed to be used. They don't have to work any more, and if you don't use muscles, you lose them!

What happens next is that about two or three weeks later, usually when you think your knee joint appears to be a lot healthier as a result of wearing the support of a knee brace, you take it off. And guess what? The pain and swelling comes back a few days later – only this time it's likely to be worse because your knee muscles are now in a worse state than they were three weeks ago. In reality, nothing has improved. Your knee support will go back over and from then on, it's a self-perpetuating cycle. Wear the support and it feels a bit easier, but your knee gets even more unhealthy. Don't wear your knee support and you suffer immediate pain or swelling. And so it rolls on.

So what do you do? The complete opposite of wearing that knee support, which is to work those knee joint muscles by doing the right exercise. So, my tip when it comes to knee or back supports is this: they are OK in the short term, and fine to wear if you're going on holiday, want to take a long walk and your knee is playing up, feeling achy or sore, OR you're recovering from a knee injury. But resist the temptation to be wearing a support all day long. That's only going to make things worse in the end.

If you could just take some time out of your day to work on a few simple strength exercises, then you would be giving your knee its own natural strength back, which, in the long run, is a lot better for your knees than any paid-for support can ever be. It might take a little bit of work, but it is the right way to help yourself to suffer from less knee pain.

Take a walk without shoes

The easiest way to protect your knee joints when you're walking or running is to make sure your footwear is comfortable, has appropriate cushioning to absorb shock and is suitable for the activity you're doing (such as running or walking). But now I'd like to introduce you to a new theory that is slowly but surely beginning to gather momentum in the fitness industry that might just change the way some people keep fit and stay healthy. Before I explain what it is, please note that I'm not advocating that you do this, I just want you to know about it, as it might help you understand some more about how to protect your knee joints.

How would you feel about walking or running in your *bare feet*? As in, without any shoes or socks on at all? It's called 'barefoot running'. Although some runners are doing it right now, it is still something that many runners and medical professionals are sceptical of. But it's worth talking about. And now I've told you about it, I guarantee that you will all of a sudden notice a lot of people doing it. Better than that, hopefully you'll find it quite interesting too, when you realise that running barefoot actually encourages your body's natural gait – the running and walking technique we were all born with and the way we were originally designed to get around.

I class it as a healthy habit because running or walking barefoot, or with minimalist footwear, is more likely to strengthen your feet than if you are wearing shoes. It is also better for your knees, because it offers a more natural way to run.

Let me explain how. Think of having to wear a knee support or a plaster cast for a month or so. When you take that support or cast away, the muscles around your knee would be weak – there's no escaping that. It happens because muscles get lazy when they don't have to work and will inevitably lose strength. When this happens, there's less support for joints coming from these muscles, meaning bones rub together MORE, and when they do, it can bring on something nasty - like osteoarthritis.

Besides that, wearing shoes on your feet is less tactile, so you're less aware of the pounding and impact, or even how hard you plant your foot each time you take a step on a hard surface. Over time, the constant heavy pounding as your foot lands during the walking or running cycle is going to take its toll. And it's not just in your ankle or foot area, as you might expect. There are also going to be problems in your knees, hips and lower back joints, which bear the brunt when your feet land hard. Have a think about the way it feels when you nip outside, say to fetch something from the car, and don't bother to put your shoes on. Think how aware you are of where you place your feet, and how slowly you do it, compared to making the same dash to your car with a pair of shoes on, and you'll get an idea what I mean when I say that not much consideration goes into how heavily you land your feet when you have shoes on.

That's why barefoot running works for runners, and is a healthier habit than running in an old pair of shoes. It puts less pressure on knee joints, because you won't be landing so hard. You will likely learn a better way of running and walking, and because of that you'll use less energy, so you'll feel better for it too. You'll even save money on replacing shoes every six months!

I agree that it might be a bit difficult to adapt to this if you're over 50 or so, because your walking habits are already formed and might be difficult to change. If you are going to give barefoot running or walking a try, my advice is to take it slow at first, focusing hard on every step. Why? Because as a result of you relying upon wearing shoes for however many years, your feet and ankle joints will be very weak. It will take you months to build up the necessary strength to run safely as fast and for as long as you can currently do wearing trainers. But, after a while, the theory is that your feet - and the rest of your body - will be stronger than ever before – which means you will be much healthier too.

If you'd like to know more about the best ways to ease knee pain, please visit my website at www.paulgoughphysio.com/knee-pain. There's a free report titled '**How to stop daily annoying and irritating knee pain WITHOUT taking painkillers, injections or bothering the GP'.** It contains all my best tips for ending knee pain naturally.

Chapter Five

Exercising simply and safely, and feeling healthy doing it

....

For the next few pages I want to show you that you don't have to use any fancy machinery or the latest keep-fit gadgets to keep yourself healthy and exercise regularly. After reading this next section, you might even decide you don't need to have that gym membership any more either!

One thing you should know about me is that I'm not the kind of physio whose head is turned by shiny new technology that hasn't got a track record of giving my clients positive results. I rarely use any machines to assist recovery. I prefer to work out a full recovery strategy for my clients that is put into play by using my hands and some good old-fashioned techniques that I know for sure work, rather than fall for the latest exercise craze or choose a new machine that promise lots of benefits, but often turns out to be a big fat letdown.

I do that because I made a point a few years ago of making sure that no money would ever change hands for healthcare where someone else could just go out and buy the solution – as in a machine – because there's no speciality if others can buy it too, and I only dispense advice or offer solutions that can solve people's specific problems. Sure, some people come looking for machines (like ultrasound or laser therapy) that I haven't got, but I made a decision to be the kind of physio who could be everything to the right someone, rather than attempting to offer something for everyone but not really helping anyone. The latter, in my humble opinion, is happening too much in healthcare these days and is contributing to the ineffectiveness of much of it, leaving lots of people more unhealthy than they should be.

So, with low-tech, easy-to-find and easy-to-use equipment in mind, and to prove to you how simple it can be to make valuable improvements to your health, here are 6 non-tech tools I regularly recommend to my clients when asked about ways to exercise that don't involve needing a gym membership.

1) A beach ball – OK, it's really called an exercise ball and you see lots of them in the gyms these days. My tip for you is to find a medium-size exercise ball, blow it up, then sit on it for about 30 seconds at a time (10 times per day) and begin to work on the core muscles of your lower back. Do this, and you will see a difference, with less backache and stiffness.

2) A Resistance Band - take a look on Amazon.com and you'll see that these multi-coloured exercise training bands are often in the top 10 best sellers list anywhere in the world. That's because they are great for improving muscle tone and control and developing the latter is the easiest way to avoid muscle pain or tension.

3) A notepad and pencil – what doesn't get written down can't be measured. And if it isn't being measured, it isn't worth doing. You must track progress or set health goals by marking them down.

4) Skipping rope – great for restoring balance after something like a knee or ankle sprain.

5) Pillow – stuff it behind the small of your back when you sit for long periods. Do this and it will improve your posture, which means you will look healthier and feel healthier, and with that, reduce stress and tension on your back muscles.

6) The bottom step of a set of stairs – this is great for building up knee strength and control. If you're suffering with something like arthritis of your knees, doing simple, low-level and non-impact exercises at the bottom of your stairs will save you the cost of having to go to a gym, yet reduce the chance of unwanted pain and stiffness.

Now, don't get me wrong, progress is a must, particularly in healthcare, and I'm not saying that all machines are fads. Just be careful not to overlook the basics and over-complicate exercise methods, because this often makes it much more difficult to stick to them. Besides, it's doing the BASICS everyday that will make the difference to your health in the long run, not how complicated or trendy whatever you're doing seems to be at the time.

When was the last time you could touch your toes?

OK, now let's talk about 'flexibility'. It's your ability to stretch and the ease with which you can freely move or bend. Without some degree of flexibility, life can be a bit more difficult than you might like and if you're 50 or over, you're probably already beginning to lose it on a daily basis. As you do begin to lose flexibility in muscles and joints (have you tried touching your toes lately?) you'll notice increasing difficulty with the simplest of things, such as putting socks and shoes on, getting in and out of the car without a struggle and even doing some household chores. And those next day aches and pains, the ones you feel after an active day spent walking or doing things in the garden, are caused by lack of flexibility too. So if it's affecting your life in any of these ways, it might help to know a little bit about it why it's happening and what you can do about it.

The big problem is this: not many people are open to the idea that you can increase your flexibility. It's as if stiffness and a lack of freedom of choice when it comes to movement are an inevitable age thing. And sure, they are – to some degree! But doesn't mean that you can't slow down these effects, or even reverse them. So here's the big question: how do you go about reducing the impact of muscles and joints getting stiffer and tighter by the day?

It's really simple: don't stop! Because the temptation is to think that because you're feeling tighter and stiffer, you should stop and wait for the stiffness to go. More often than not, that's the worst thing you can do, and rarely does it do anything other than get worse. Swimming, bike riding and walking are all fabulous ways of preventing flexibility problems in your 50s and 60s – even if you only do each one for 30-40 minutes, three times a week. And here's a way to get some added benefits of being active: When you finish doing any of these things, before you drop back on the couch, stretch a few of the muscles you usually have the problems with. At this point, after a nice run, swim, walk or ride around town, your body is in the best state it can possibly be to be stretched out, because it is warm. It's so much easier and safer to stretch muscles and joints when you're warm.

My own routine is often to stretch at the halfway mark, and then again at the end of my bike ride or run. I'll find a nice place to pull over (preferably with a nice view to enjoy whilst I'm doing it), and stretch all my shoulder, back and leg muscles for about 10-15 minutes. It feels great when I'm done! Another way you could improve you flexibility is to find a yoga class - and attend it regularly.

While I'm on the subject, let's talk some more about yoga – because it's my humble opinion that it's one of the best habits you could ever have. Let me tell you a nice story and at the same time, give you some more information about yoga.

The health benefits of regular yoga

My attention was caught when I happened to hear 'Namaste Yoggies!' over the very loud PA system booming around the park. A 2500+ gathering of men, women and children were taking part in a very relaxing and great for your health open-air yoga class. A hot one too. It was 90 degrees plus in Grants Park, Central Chicago where I happened to be that particular weekend. I was there talking at a fitness industry seminar when I stumbled upon this epic yoga class.

Without knowing you personally, I'm not sure what you

even think about yoga, but I'm sure you have heard of it. It's true that yoga is more popular and much better attended in the big cities around the UK. I can even understand how people might suggest it's just a fad, a trendy thing to do, but really, it isn't. It's just a really healthy activity to do once or twice per week. If you've never thought about giving it a try, I'd strongly urge you to consider it.

Here's why: It's a simple exercise routine that you can quickly learn to do on your own. Even just doing 20 minutes per day of the stretching and posture exercises involved will see a significant and positive difference in how healthy you look and feel. And if you're aged 50 or above, I'd go so far as to say there's nothing more important that you should be doing on a daily basis than a progressive programme of stretching exercises such as the ones you'll learn at yoga. Not a lot of people know this, but every day you wake up, you're actually getting a little stiffer and a tiny bit smaller, so by continuously stretching these muscles out by doing yoga, you're actively doing something to counteract those bad things happening to you. Getting smaller and tighter on a daily basis is not something you'll notice each day, but over time, it is creeping up on us all. And doing yoga is one of the best ways to combat it. It makes your muscles more flexible, your joints more supple and importantly, you're less likely to suffer from things like neck and shoulder pain, lower back pain, hamstring injuries and even Achilles pain.

Agreed, it might look a bit strange... and at first it might even feel a bit strange, but for most people who do it, once they've done it for six weeks, that's it - they're hooked on how great doing it regularly makes them feel. I can say from my own experience that if I do it first thing in the morning, my whole day seems to be that much easier. Some people like to do it at night and that's healthy too because it makes you feel very relaxed and almost guarantees a good night's sleep.

Why don't you give it a go and see how you get on? There aren't many people who won't benefit from doing it, so chances are you will. All you have to do is show up and follow the instructor for a few weeks, and then you can begin to make it a daily habit once you learn a few techniques.

The best time to do yoga

Between 30 and 40, recovery from physical activity begins to take that little bit longer. As the post-exercise aches and pains become more noticeable, particularly the next morning, doing yoga is going to make a positive difference to the speed at which you will recover from playing golf, walking with friends, being in the garden or playing five-a-side football – even cleaning the house. Doing regular yoga stretches will dramatically affect the flexibility and control of your muscles – in a good way. That's because yoga acts like a counterbalance to your muscles' shortening and ensures that when needed, they will flex and stretch safely. This will hugely reduce your chances of becoming injured in the first place. It also means that the muscles will return to their original length more quickly after exercise and when this happens, you'll get fewer next-day aches and pains.

To understand this better, think how it feels when you take a long walk for the first time in a while, or spend the first day of spring in the garden after a few months of being absent from it - inevitably the next day can be pretty tough with muscles feeling stiff and tight and your body just generally achy. This happens because muscles have been stretched further than they have been used to in a while. That pain the next day is these muscles shortening after the blood supply has stopped and not wanting to move until your body can work out a way to help them relax.

The theory behind yoga is that it improves your breathing, control and balance and aims to make all the muscles you're likely to use during physical activity more efficient, saving you energy and helping you feel healthier as a result. Improving balance reduces injury and if your muscles are working more efficiently, they are likely to produce less of the nasty substances such as lactic acid (a chemical released in your system after exercise) which can contribute to that next-day soreness too.

If you do begin to start a few yoga routines, it's important for you to understand that <u>little and often</u> is more beneficial than doing a lot occasionally, and that your progress is going to be slow. You may not feel or see any difference for months – but it will be starting to work. So don't walk away at the end of your first class and expect immediate changes, because it isn't going to happen.

A bum like Pippa Middleton's - Pilates

The reality of being healthy as you hope to be, staying active for as long as you can and having your body in good enough condition to let you do all you want to do when you want to do it is that it does take some effort on your part. There's no getting away from it. I honestly believe that most people know they need to do something to make themselves physically fitter or more active, they're just a bit confused about what to do for the best. If that's you, I have a suggestion for you to consider: it's joint first on my list of ways to reduce the aches and pains associated with growing graciously older every day. It's called Pilates.

Pilates, done on a regular basis, will improve the control and tone of your muscles. If you do that you'll reduce the chances of suffering from back pain or shoulder muscle pain or tension, and if you improve your muscle tone, it will help you to look more healthy too.

Which would be a nice added bonus, right? And the best thing about Pilates - it's really simple to do, once you know how. I recommend it to clients all the time, especially those with lower back pain and problems in the neck and shoulder area.

The theory is that if the core muscle group which wraps around your lower back is made stronger and more in control of the joints down there, your risk of injury reduces hugely and with it so does the amount of stiffness or tension you will suffer each day.

Your lower back is the powerhouse of your body - if it is strong and healthy, then the chances are most other parts of your body will be strong and healthy too. On the flip side, if your lower back is weak, then it's likely you will suffer from stiffness, constant aches and pains and maybe even be left feeling tired all the time. Although I view Pilates as one of the best and most significant advances in exercise science in the last twenty years, it has in fact been around for hundreds of years. A guy called Joseph Pilates invented it, and its popularity is gathering momentum as more people cotton on to how important it can be to improving their health – especially now that we're all now sitting a lot more than we were ever designed to (which is not good if you want a healthy, pain-free lower back).

Thanks to some new, healthier ways of thinking, and to people like Pippa Middleton who put Pilates in the news back at the time of the Royal Wedding in 2012 - she said she had such a widely-admired bum because she does Pilates regularly - it's becoming a lot more popular and mainstream, particularly with ladies aged 40, 50 and 60. Ever since that wedding we've seen a huge increase in the number of ladies asking us about Pilates. Before the wedding, it was nearly always us asking them if they had tried it.

So, Pilates is something I'd urge you to seriously consider looking into. Again, like yoga, you could find a class, go along for a few months and learn the routines, then begin to adopt a few of them yourself at home and even start your own exercise class – on your front room floor!

So what actually is Pilates? It's a simple set of control exercises done in sequence, and most classes last about 40-45 minutes. Doing it regularly is going to ease muscle tension in your neck and shoulders, limit back pain, make you look much healthier when you begin to stand up tall with your shoulders back (not rounded and protruding forwards as most people do), and, as an added bonus, it's done to soothing music and is very relaxing too. So, it's great for the mind and body and that's got to be a healthy bonus, right?

Want proof of how important Pilates style exercises are to keeping you healthy and active? At my private physiotherapy practice I employ a specialist physiotherapy

Pilates instructor who designs and crafts exercise programmes for my clients with 80% of the routines involving those you might find in a Pilates exercise hall. That means that when our clients come and visit us, as well as giving them hands-on care like the massage and skilled joint techniques to get tight muscles and joints moving, we give each client a specially-designed Pilates exercise workout plan to take home and start to work on that same night. The transformations in health we hear about from our clients doing these routines often happen within weeks, and clients tell us of seeing (and feeling) stunning improvements in their posture, not forgetting a significant reduction in things like back and shoulder muscle pain.

My tip: Find a reputable instructor and go along to a class just once a week. Then simply add 5-10 minutes of Pilates-style exercises to the beginning and end of your day. If your children are able to do it with you, why not make it a family routine?

Why so many people are unhappy or bored at work

Let me ask you this: What's your ultimate goal in wanting to keep fit? Or even, how come you're reading this book in the first place? Sure, it might be to find one or two tips to help keep you more active and healthier, but when you really think about it, isn't the ultimate reason that all of us try to find more of both is so that we can add something to our levels of happiness?

Here's what I mean: The more research I do on health and fitness, the more references to happiness I'm finding. There are lessons in being unhappy in life, that can be taken across to your attempt to stay active and healthy. The reality of most people's unhappiness is that it stems from boredom. And by that I mean that most people aren't unhappy - they're just bored!

Think about any job you ever disliked, or perhaps the job you're currently disliking going to every day. It's probably happening because the role lacks novelty, surprise or any opportunity to do new things. The excitement of what was once a job you enjoyed, even loved, has vanished. Yet the job and its requirements remain exactly the same. In essence, nothing's changed! And that's the real problem people should to face up to before they spend years grumbling about their working situation.

One of the many misconceptions about happiness is the idea that if everything just stays the same as it is now, you will be happy for the rest of your days. You work so hard to get into a new job or a new relationship (or out of one), and it's common to think that those first exciting few months are how you will always feel. But that's not possible. Even if things do stay the same, you'll never be as happy as you were at first. Apart from the joy and happiness that comes from your children, it's just not possible for feelings to stay the same way, and it's all because of chemicals in your body that make you adapt to the environment you're in every day.

And you know what? I see many people around me suffering from this way of thinking and feeling – friends, family, colleagues and clients included. It's very easy for us to fall into the trap of trying to control our lives, never shifting from what we know works, just so we can try and stay as happy as we know now - not wanting to risk ever being happier, just in case we're left feeling unhappier.

When you know this is happening to you, it's much easier to override it. It's the reason why I sometimes love to do what appear to others to be quite random things, like travel to third world countries on a whim, make more effort to talk to new people who I don't know and am never likely to meet again, try new outdoor adventure sports and even employ new staff who are nothing like any others that I've got around me each day – just to work with some different people. It's also the reason why I devoted a whole chapter to it earlier on.

For most people as they live their lives, the reality is that they're not as eager to do new things as someone like me, and I always respect that. The problem is, not wanting to try new things can seriously impact people's health – and I find that a lot more difficult to ignore!

It's true that doing the unfamiliar and the unexpected have been proven to bring great happiness. I accept that it might be a jump to far to want to spontaneously change jobs or careers every other week if you are unhappy. That, of course, would be reckless. But, given that happiness can be found just by doing something unfamiliar or unexpected, what's stopping anyone from changing their exercise routines once in a while and trying something new in an attempt to bring more of it (happiness)? Nothing, when you really think about it!

Besides, as I wrote earlier, doing the same exercise routine night after night is not good for your joints or your muscles. So there are two very good reasons for changing a routine or varying the exercise you do – one physical, one psychological, but both PROVEN to make you happier and healthier. So why do people insist on doing the same thing when it comes to exercise? Quite simply because they feel safer doing so. It was OK yesterday, they felt good for doing it then, so they think that if they just keep doing it, they'll keep feeling good about it tomorrow and every day after that. But as I mentioned earlier in this section, you can't possibly continue to feel the same level of happiness from the same source, so it's in your best interests to mix it up with new things like yoga and Pilates, or even a gentle jog or a weekly swim.

And with that in mind, here's something for you...

Tips for beginners when starting to exercise

Let's imagine you're thinking about increasing the amount of exercise or activity you do. You like the sound of yoga and Pilates, but you're going to play it safe with a few very gentle walks, or maybe even a jog. Here are a few things you should consider.

The number one most important thing when doing any exercise is your choice of footwear. Trainers don't need to be all that expensive, but don't under estimate the importance of a decent pair of running or walking shoes. Tennis shoes won't do, the trendy white plimsolls are definitely out and resist the temptation to choose those old tired running shoes you've occasionally used over the past few years that are currently stuffed away in the cupboard somewhere. Yes, to reduce the risk of aches and pains in muscles and damage to your joints from the pounding they take off the hard street surfaces, you'll be better off in fresh, well-cushioned running or walking shoes. After all, running shoes are designed for running and if you're a beginner, your legs are going to need all the protection they can get. My advice, if you're buying, is don't go for the obvious big name brands either - they might look great, maybe even match your outfit, but they are not always what you need to protect joints.

Please know this too: each brand of trainer such as Nike, or Adidas etc, will have its own instep shape for your foot to fit into - and they can't all be right for yours, it's just not possible. So, once you've found the brand or style that works best for you, the one that feels comfortable and lets you walk or run without any major issues, stick with it! I've seen injuries like shin splints and Achilles tendon problems happen simply because a client has swapped the make or manufacturer of the trainers they wear.

Here's another tip: Wear something comfortable. Most new (and naive) runners will overdress at the beginning, forgetting how hot they will quickly become. It takes just 6-7 minutes to get your body warm and believe it or not there is a metric you can follow when it comes to the amount of clothing you should be wearing. It goes like this: If the temperature is +12 Celsius, shorts and a tee shirt or vest will do. If the temperature drops below 8 Celsius or you're a very early morning runner, step up to leggings and a long sleeve tee shirt. Now, if the temperature drops below that, personally, I like to run wearing my hat and gloves. Why? Well, it's because hands take the longest to warm up and it's argued that heat is lost through your head. So, it's better to have the warm blood supply hitting the important muscles you're going to be using, such as the ones in your legs, than it being directed to your hands, which are pretty un-important in the grand scheme of things.

The importance of a varied exercise regime

OK, so far in this chapter I've introduced you to things like Pilates and yoga. Then I showed you some secret tips for starting to ease into running or becoming a frequent walker. Next, let's talk about good old-fashioned swimming and see if we can add this to your routine, too. The reason why swimming is important? There are enough good ones to fill a book, and that's why swimming is on my top 5 list of the best and safest ways to exercise and keep healthy.

Doing it *often* can have a dramatic effect on lowering blood pressure levels, particularly if you're 60 or over. Not long ago now, I read a study about swimming which revealed that those who swim three times per week have a chance of significantly lowering their systolic blood pressure reading significantly. Not sure what that is? Well, it's the most important one – the one where your GP would be happy to see a low number rather than a high one. Simply, it's the rate at which your heart is beating when it rests. The results of the study acted as an important reminder that there are many options available for people to exercise, no matter what their age or the state of things like their knees or hips - as there aren't many people who can't get in a pool and do a few lengths.

People often associate exercising with running, cycling, even walking. Yet swimming is possibly the best way of all, simply because it's easy on the joints and not likely to cause much overheating of your body, as the cold water is going to cool you down. Here are some more benefits of swimming: 1) it's something you can do on your own, 2) you don't have to worry about the dark nights or pairing up with someone to stay safe (as you might do with running) and 3) it's relatively inexpensive for the health benefits you get. More: one of the biggest benefits of swimming, particularly for the 50+ age group, is that the buoyancy of the water makes it friendly to ankle, knee and back joints because there's almost none of the stress or impact which might happen if you were walking or running.

Confessions of a physio who didn't take his own advice

I couldn't finish this section on the importance of varying your activity and exercise routines without telling you this true story. At the time of writing, I'd been struggling with a foot injury. I'd like to tell you a bit more about it and show how you can stop something similar happening to you.

Here goes… So I love to keep active. For me, sitting in the house isn't really an option and my home is more like a hotel because all I ever use it for is to sleep in at night. And, because I'm happy to say that I'm addicted (no exaggeration) to the feeling that I get from exercising *daily*, sometimes I do too much and my body hurts as a result. And this particular summer, because of wanting to spend more playtime after work with my little boy (Harry), I became what I call a lazy runner. What I mean by that is that I had succumb to the temptation to quickly and easily go for a run most nights after work so that I could get back and spend more time playing with him on the floor in our big (Disney themed) toy room.

I paid the price! I got in my right foot the beginnings of what could have led to a stress fracture, no doubt caused by my pounding the streets of Hartlepool a few too many times in succession. When I noticed it, and only when I grew concerned, I stopped the running and got back on my bike a lot more, and even found time to get to the local swimming pool.

Because riding my bike takes about 90 minutes to get the same feeling as a 30-minute jog (plus prep time to find clothing, helmet, fill up water bottles etc), I had to seriously re-engineer my day so I could still see Harry before his Mam enforces his 8.30 pm bed time. And guess what? Because I spent so much time in the sitting position and riding my bike nearly every night, I developed a lot of tension and discomfort in both shoulders – don't ask me why, but the left one was worse. I remember thinking that it felt like my posture was awkward too, with my shoulders rounded, and I was definitely suffering a lot of stiffness in my lower back as well.

So the moral of the story is this: If you run a lot, expect

problems to surface somewhere, like your foot or your shins. If you cycle a lot, shoulder and lower back problems WILL occur. And it's not just these two types of activities that come with some health risks either. Take golf for example - I see golfers in my clinic regularly and they nearly always come in with an Achilles tendon problem, or a lower back issue. And what about if you play bowls? Well, a bad knee (or two) is common. Hill or fell walking? Same as the golfers, lower back and Achilles injuries.

Even swimmers – the one activity you might think is REALLY good for you (which it is) is still going to cause physical problems with your shoulders and neck from the repetitive nature of arms swinging forward with your neck constantly being held out of the water (a reason to wear goggles is so that you don't have to suffer this) – if you did it every day. Do you want to know the solution? Great, here it is: read back to the beginning of this section (and through this chapter) and you'll realise that the REAL root cause of own my own health issues was not from me biking or running. No. It was due to my insistence on NOT planning my day properly to find the time to vary my exercise. At times, maybe we're all guilty of thinking we don't have the *time* to do things properly and it's only human nature to try and find a short cut to do something quicker – even if it's our health at stake! But, like as you've just read in this story, isn't it true that when pain strikes, all of a sudden it's pretty easy to re-work your day to find time to do the one thing you should have been doing in the first place? If you're guilty of it, I assure you you're not alone.

So, with that story firmly at the front of your mind, here's what I want you to take away from this chapter: one of the best bits of advice I could ever give to you if you are considering taking part in any type of increased exercise programme (or activity) is to *constantly vary your activity*. Now you've got yoga, Pilates, walking, jogging, and you can add some swimming in there too. Mix any of these and you'll dramatically lower the chance of repetitive strain type injuries from happening to you.

A timely, important note: Anyone taking part in any form of increased exercise should always check with their GP. But more and more studies are pointing towards swimming as being as safe as walking and bike-riding when it comes to looking at a way to improve your cardio-vascular health. Please check with your GP first that it's safe for you to do so.

Chapter Six

Healthy habits and daily rituals

■■■■■■■■■■■■■■

This next chapter is all about you finding some very healthy habits and daily rituals that are going to make a positive difference in your life. But first, let's go back to you being 30. And, here's my question to you: Are your thirties the BEST years of your life?

It's a question that a very valued client of mine (named Bridget), posed to me on the day of my 30th birthday. Truth be told, she TOLD me they were. And the reason why was this:

It's the time of your life when you have just the right mix of wisdom and life experience, and you have great physical health to enjoy it. Yet, as you hit 40, the pendulum tips in favour of you having more wisdom and experience, and your physical health somewhat begins to falter. And from then on, you're acquiring more wisdom and knowledge, but you're not always able to get out and enjoy it because you're health doesn't always allow.

So, what do you think? Would you agree with Bridget?

Here's the thing: At some point in life, usually round the age of 30, every person wakes up one Monday morning with aches and pains that weren't there the day before. Doing a simple bit of DIY, a spot of gardening or even just a standard game of five-a-side with workmates could have easily caused those aches and pains and it's usually a good indicator that you've tipped 30. In your workplace or even in your home, it's probably going to be called 'getting old' and if you let slip that you're stiff or achy it doesn't take long before one of your work colleagues or even a family member delights in that fact that you've tipped the other side of 30.

Now it's not for me to say whether or not your thirties are indeed the best years of your life, but I am allowed to say that they are DEFINITELY the time of your life when things like physical activity and exercising start to take just that little bit longer to get over or recover from. Why do you think the world's top athletes and sportsmen always seem to reach their peak of performance in their twenties?

Now some people choose to grow old gracefully, bowing out of being active, exercising and playing sport at the first sign of aches and pains in muscles that seem now to take DAYS to recover from. But some people battle on and choose to continue with things like Sunday morning football, golf, cricket and even running with a club well into their 50s and 60s. And that's in spite of the aches, pains and stiffness that are inevitably suffered in muscles and joints for two or three days after.

And that's great! You know those aches and pains you get after activity - the ones where your Achilles or calf muscles feel so tight when you first get out of bed on a morning it feels like your foot doesn't want to move, and even if it does, it's going to hurt. They are actually very normal. But they come with accepting that the optimum period for physical activity was in your twenties. In your twenties you're able to do pretty much anything physical without the consequence of suffering for days after. Was it also in your early thirties that you realised that the hangovers took an extra day or so to get over, too?

Now, some of these natural changes confuse a lot of people I talk too – they just can't figure out what to do about them. So, with that in mind, I'll talk through this topic a bit more.

At EVERY stage of your life, you're going through a natural ageing process that just means it takes that little bit longer for muscles to return to their normal size. You see, at first, all muscles are very flexible and elastic. Ever watched a baby sleep and wonder how they can get into such positions with legs underneath and arms wrapped round their head? It's because muscles and joints are so flexible at that age. But as you grow older by the day, these muscles become less flexible and are not only more prone to injury, but take much longer to return to their normal length. So whenever you stretch these muscles, say, playing tennis, badminton, cycling, a round of golf, going for a run, or even just doing the gardening, you're actually stretching them muscles beyond a limit that is slowly but surely reducing everyday as you age.

To sum up: In your twenties, you're king. You're able to do to pretty much any type of exercise, activity or sport, any time you like. Then, as you move into your thirties, it's about accepting that in order to prolong your participation in exercise or any form of physical activity, you might have to occasionally pick your battles. And, by that I mean being more selective in when and how you're going to be active and keep yourself fit.

I'm about to say something again that I've already spoken about a few times in this book: the key is to vary your activity by doing things like yoga, Pilates, swimming, bike riding and even brisk walking. That way you'll be keeping your muscles and joints as supple and as flexible as possible, no matter what phase of life you're in.

Who else felt washed up at 40?

Now, let's skip ahead 10 years and talk about being 40. The problems really are definitely more noticeable now. This is when many people begin some kind of relationship with a physio. Experiencing a spike in the amount of aches and pains and even injuries like sciatica, Achilles tendon pain or neck joint problems is not uncommon. In fact, they're more likely to happen to you in this age bracket than at any other time of your life. Here's why.

As you've just read, earlier in your life, say when you're in your twenties, your body is the most flexible and strongest it's ever likely to be. So as you're running around doing everyday things like shopping, lifting the children in and out of the car, keeping fit, doing the housework and driving to and from work, the strength and flexibility you have in these early decades of your life, is easily able to absorb all of this physical stress that you place on your body.

Yet as you now know, somewhere around the age of 40, your flexibility starts to decline. And it usually happens fast! For some people, it literally happens overnight! Maybe it felt like that was what happened to you? And, I'd say this losing the ability to move as easily or as freely as you once could is one of the major consequences of growing older. Yes, the muscles and joints that were once able to cope with just about anything you wanted to do, all of a sudden, can't. And it's because they're shrinking and shortening.

How come? Well, think of your muscles as elastic bands getting pulled tighter and tighter, slowly but surely more each day. Without getting scientific, your muscles lose flexibility because they are repeatedly being used, even damaged. Although it's not the kind of damage you ever know much about, just using them every day is enough to produce micro damage to muscles which, over time, builds and causes problems. And to repair this micro damage, your body uses something called collagen - you might know it as scar tissue (I call it glue) - to repair these muscles.

But, this stuff is NOT very elastic or flexible. And is why at 40, when you've got loads of it in your muscles, you really start to feel less flexible. This lack of flexibility in your muscles is happening at a time when you're still very active, too. And because of that, it's a hot spot time for injuries.

Now think of what life is like, or will be like, in your 60s. The lack of flexibility and strength issue is still happening, but your daily activities and physical demands are likely to be much less than they were in your 40s and 50s. So the stress you're placing on these muscles and tendons is not as much, meaning less chance of problems such as back and knee pain (or general next-day aches and pains). The solution? You guessed it - regular and sustained attendance at a yoga and or Pilates class. Both of these are perfect to make muscles more flexible and give them back some much needed tone and control which is going to protect your joints. Last thing: If you're experiencing more and more stiffness in places like your back, shoulders or Achilles, then these two classes are something that you might wish to consider, as they will help reduce it.

Housework and waistlines

Next, let's talk about some daily habits that might be able to keep you healthy and active. This first one may even be able to help you shed a few pounds (it might not be needed, of course!)

Doing housework has the ability to delight, frustrate or anger you and as well as all of those feelings, it can even cause physical injury. Yes - some of the most common and simple injuries that I see in my physio practice occur as a result of someone trying relentlessly to maintain a clean and tidy house. But let me ask you this: have you ever considered that housework might be a legitimate addition to a weekly exercise routine? And another question: is a vigorous spring clean (where you REALLY go at the house) capable of reducing your waistline, if you were ever looking to trim it? Interested to know more? Read on...

I've heard it said by many ladies that housework is their best form of exercise. But here's something to consider: as the years have progressed, it seems housework and waistlines are heading in opposite directions and doing the housework isn't as good for you as it once was. Why? It's because of things like slim line and lighter vacuum cleaners, the average family not being as big as it was a few decades ago, and new, more advanced cleaning products designed to make scrubbing easier. All these mean you're not likely to be burning as many calories as you might have thought (or hoped) or once did.

As a general rule of thumb, the experts predict that you can burn up to 200 calories with a typical one-hour clean of an average-sized house. To put that into context, if you see somebody out jogging, hoping to burn some off fat off, that person running is going to have to keep going for 20-25 minutes just to match the same calorie burn as you'll be getting from doing your house clean. So as you look to keep active, maybe even trim down, bear in mind there's an alternative to going to the gym. Keeping your house ultra clean and tidy can provide the very strong incentive of reducing your waistline at the same time. It can still produce the feel-good chemicals that you experience after a power walk or run. But, here's one final thing to consider: two hundred calories burned might sound great - and it is - but now picture yourself after finishing your cleaning with your feet up (shoes off, of course), on your freshly-cleaned couch with a nice, hard-earned glass of wine in hand and watching your favourite soap on TV - you've just put all those 200 calories back on in an instant!

How to stay out of Fat Club

Let's stay on the topic of weight loss. In my clinic and with my office staff, it's nearly always a hot topic of conversation. And there's lots of confusion, dangerous half-truths and even myths about the best ways to avoid getting, or feeling, or actually being, fat! Would you like to know some hard-hitting truths about this topic? You do? Good!

So, about getting fat… the rule is this: it's affected 80% by what you eat, and how active you are accounts for only 20% of what fat remains in your body. And if looking slim and trim is your goal, those are just one of many facts that you need to know about. Another is the daily average calorie intake you're allowed to consume before you will get fat (or fatter), which is approximately 2500 for men, 2000 for a woman. Go over that limit for a few too many days on the trot and you will get fat! Simple.

If you don't want to get fat, you're also going to need two more things. One is discipline and the other is an understanding that whatever diet you choose - and remember that you are choosing your own diet with every decision over what YOU choose to consume - it must be sustainable. That is, you must be able to keep it up for more than a week (the latter being why most people fall off their diets).

Summer is the time when most people are more aware of their weight. After a long winter of eating chocolate and heavy meals to warm you up, combined with dark nights and sitting on the couch, just about everyone wants to be trim for summer, usually so they can fit into their nice clothes or wear less of them. True? OK, picture a time when you're coming back from a holiday. Chances are on the flight on the way home you were already thinking about starting a diet - knowing how hard it's going to be to lose the pounds you've just so easily enjoyed putting on.

But here's the thing: if you are ever going to go on a diet, sustainability is crucial and you should always be asking this question: *will I be able to keep this diet up for a long time?* That's the one and only thing you should be ramming down your neck when considering a diet.

I have two girls in my office and they are both regularly in and out of weight loss clubs. If you ask me, they look fabulously healthy as it is - but I guess it's each to their own. The one thing I point out to both, even when they come in pleased as punch about how many pounds they've lost this week at fat club (their words, not mine), is this: can you sustain whatever it is that is causing the weight to drop off? And if they answer no, then I tell them to forget the whole thing, because it's a short-term pleasure that will bring more false hope than anything else. Here's what I mean: how many times have you been on a diet, sacrificed lots of situations where you might have been able to enjoy a nice meal or an evening out with friends, all for the pleasure rush of losing a few pounds, just to look better? Sure, you might have achieved it, but how long before you suffered the disappointment of the flab coming back, just a few weeks after going back to your old eating habits?

You know what, if you're not careful, weight loss can become a fallacy. And a lifelong one at that. Worse - the satisfaction of losing a few pounds once in a while will never last as long as the disappointment you feel when you put them all back on. So be careful not to let it become an impossible dream that you're forever chasing. If you're faced with losing some pounds to protect your health on the advice of a GP, follow it like your life depends upon it. And do it with a simple diet that is sustainable. That means working out what calories are in what foods and then doing some basic maths - every day. If you hit your limit, you're done for the day! And if you hit the limit, but really can't resist, then you need to be disciplined enough to go for a nice long walk or swim to burn off the excess.

Maybe think of it like this: once every other week, wherever you live, you get to put your bins out. If the contents of the bin overflow, you're unlikely to stand there and continue ramming more rubbish into it. That would be nuts! Because, if your bin men are anything like mine, by now you know that they won't take it anyway! So the excess rubbish will get left on your drive. This is no different from what happens to your stomach, bum and chin. Go over your calorie intake and your body, like the bin men, can't remove it. But this time the rubbish is not getting stored on your drive - much worse than that, it's getting stored as fat, clogging up your arteries, adding pressure to your joints and leading to health problems that will arrive sooner than you hope. When it comes to weight loss, for most of us, best just to apply some basic maths.

How to enjoy a HEALTHY day in the garden

Ever heard the saying what makes you bad makes you better? Well, sometimes, what makes you feel good makes you feel bad! Want proof? OK, think about the last time you had just a bit too much alcohol. Great at the time, but I bet you were made to pay for it the very next day!

But drinking too much alcohol isn't the only thing that can cause problems the next day. Gardening can easily cause them too. Backache or pain is often an inevitable consequence of a few too many hours spent in the garden or an allotment. And in the same way that spending too long in a beer garden will cause pain in your head and stomach, gardening for hours on end is also likely to cause problems such as stiffness, nerve pain or even muscle spasms in your back and knees – and make them all much more likely to happen when you least expect them to.

But it's not the garden that's the problem. No, it's how

you're working on it, and specifically, the positions you have to get into when trying to keep it in great shape. I've learned over the years that problems caused by spending too much time in the garden are as regular as clockwork and very easy to predict. So much so that just before any summer bank holiday weekend, we often joke in our office that the phones will be on red alert when we reopen, with a flurry of over-keen gardeners wanting some attention on their lower back – which is likely to be so stiff that they can barely get out of a chair. And we're never let down!

In the same way that the sun will send people to the beer gardens for hours on end, it will also send people to their own gardens and allotments for just the same length of time. And here's the real problem with that. Gardening means you usually have to lean over or bend forwards for long periods of time (that's obvious, I know). Even something as simple as pushing a lawnmower means you're leaning just slightly forward, which isn't good for your lower back. The issue here is that in this position, your spine and the muscles surrounding it are in their most vulnerable position. Meaning they could get damaged at any time (more so than when you're sitting, too). In fact, there is almost a third more pressure on your lower back when you're in this 'leaning forward' position than when in any other. That's something to be wary of - even when you're in the kitchen cooking.

Spending time repetitively leaning forward is also the

reason why I've had so many people visit my physio clinic for back pain that came on suddenly just from leaning over the sink to brush their teeth. It might sound a really innocuous and a simple activity, but leaning forward constantly is not healthy and makes you prone to these types of problems throughout your life. Strengthening your lower back muscles is the most effective way to avoid regular back pain, and the exercise routines you would find in any good Pilates class are able to help combat this.

Wear the right clothing when you exercise

Let's talk about the dark nights. They always come around fast, and tend to dominate conversations. They impact your life and change your daily routines hugely. Apart from a lack of vitamin D – the chemicals your body creates when you're in the sun that make you feel great – the darkness also changes your exercise habits. At least, it often gives people an excuse to do so.

If you're not careful, you'll suffer the double whammy of a lack of both vitamin D and the endorphins your body produces when you're active or exercising, the real reason why people suffer the winter blues. You might be forgiven for thinking you've got that SAD syndrome (seasonal affective disorder), but in reality, no such condition exists, it's just something the media made up a few years back which gives people an excuse to be miserable! Quick question: Did you know that visitors to a physio clinic like mine suffering with lower back stiffness increase by more than 30% between October and April? It's true! And I'll explain why.

In summer, it's easy to stumble across a new love of being active, whether walking, cycling or jogging, on your own or with friends. But chances are, when the dark nights draw in, it's a lot easier to take one look out of the window at that same walk or cycle route you were taking only weeks ago – and skip it. That means you're going to end up spending much more time indoors and crucially, sitting. Sitting in your car or on the bus, sitting at work, sitting on the way home from work and now, because the weather's not quite as you fancy, six months of sitting on the couch and staring at the TV. At least that's what can happen if you're not careful.

So, what's the solution? Simple - don't change anything. The exercise routine shouldn't change. It doesn't need to. The *where* you do it, ie the sea front or local park, doesn't need to change and even the *why* you do it (to feel great and keep healthy), shouldn't. No, the only thing that needs to change is the *how* you do it. As in, what you wear to shut out the cold and damp and keep you safe in the dark.

It's just a simple case of investing in the right clothes and equipment. When it comes to the UK weather, I'm a big believer that the only difference between a good day and bad day is the clothing you're wearing. So here's a big tip: to keep active and exercising all year round, when you're finding it easy and enjoyable being active in the middle of a warm summer and you're feeling great because of the amount of exercise-induced chemicals that you've got rushing round your body, *then* is the time to start thinking about what you're going to need to invest in to keep doing it in the winter - because you'll be highly motivated to do so.

Here's a little known fact: there's lots of research that suggests that treating yourself to the right clothing or equipment will make exercising more pleasant and you more likely to sustain it, even in winter.

If you're serious about your health and you do want to keep active, consider investing just a little bit of time and money on warmer exercise clothing or reflective equipment before winter arrives to make exercising much more enjoyable and likely to happen regularly, as well as safer.

On your bike!

The health benefits of cycling are endless. For me, it's rivalled only by swimming. Doing regular cycling can help improve physical fitness, ease mental stress (with the rush of the endorphins and 'feel-great' chemicals that will be released), and it's also a great way to reduce your weight, not to mention to see some nice sights if you pick a scenic route.

If you're having regular problems with arthritic knees or hips, a really stiff lower back, or even tightness of muscles such as Achilles and calves, then cycling is a great option and you'll likely benefit from doing it more often. Even doing it for just 30 minutes or so at a time. Why? Because you'll be reducing the impact of the hard surface that can easily damage vital joints and at the same time, you're still helping essential things like your heart and lungs to stay healthy.

It's so important that I want to say it again - you'll feel a lot healthier if you vary your exercise habits and training or fitness plans and remain alert to the impact that doing the same thing night after night is having upon joints and muscles (it's nearly always negative). Bike riding is something that anyone in their 50s or above who is looking to be more active should seriously consider. It offers an alternative to pounding streets and it's even better than walking if you're objective is to stay active and healthy.

Now let's abolish a myth about bike riding: many people think that to have the same positive impact on your health as say going for a run, you have to do much more when riding a bike. I've found this confusion to be one of the most common objections when I suggest people consider taking a bike ride. It's true that to get the endorphins and the feel-great rush you're wanting from exercising, you do have to sit on your bike for a bit longer than if you were just going to head out for a run.

With that in mind, here are some facts on bike riding vs running. Someone who weighs approximately 12 stone will burn roughly 650 calories from doing an hour's bike riding. With a typical 20-minute run, you will probably be lucky to lose 200. So, although it might not feel that way, you're working just as hard, only much more safely in terms of the reduced impact on your knees and hips. Something to think about. When the numbers stack up like this, you can see why more and more people aged 50+ are getting back on their bikes to keep healthy and feel and look great.

Good habits to reduce stiffness

To wrap up this section on daily health habits, I've got a few more suggestions to show you. But first let me answer this common question about being stiff which I get asked regularly by clients of my clinic. The answer and tips I'll provide are done to help provide clarity and clear up the confusion that getting stiffer as you grow older doesn't have to come with a lack of choice. There *are* thing you can do. Anyhow, here's the question:

Paul, do you have any advice for someone like me who ISN'T in a lot of pain? I'm just incredibly stiff every day and suffering in a way that means I can't do things as easily as I would like?

With that in mind, here are four quick and easy tips to add to your daily routine that will help you find a life with less stiffness, whatever age you are:

1) Swim - daily if possible but at least twice a week. Problems like arthritis are multiplied when you stop or slow down. Swimming offers a very simple and safe way of keeping joints moving and a regular dose of moving in the water is way better than any medication or magic pills that promise joint lubrication.

2) Stretch - daily. My tip, 7 minutes on a morning when you first get up, 7 minutes on a night before bed (doing yoga just before bed can help you get a much better night's sleep, too.)

3) Avoid long periods of sitting - you're better off stretching full out on the couch than you are sitting in a chair for long periods. We're NOT designed to sit, and stretching out can be a nice relief for muscles and joints, particularly if you've had a long day spent in a chair.

4) Walk – for at least twenty minutes a day. Next time you need to make a long phone call, why not do it on your mobile and take a walk at the same time?

The sad thing is that most people accept stiffness in their life as though it's normal and nothing can be done about it. Stiffness in joints such as your lower back, neck, knees or ankles, is a warning sign that something needs to be done - **by you**. Warning: the day you accept stiffness into your life is a bad one – thereafter, it will not only remain with you, it will get worse, and quickly.

Chapter Seven

Unhealthy habits

■■■■■■■■■■■■■■

Now let's talk about the complete opposite of healthy habits – the bad ones. Because it often helps just to become aware of them - and an easy way to make improvements is to just cut them out. So here goes.

Too much coffee in the office

The golden hour in most people's lives is often on a morning when they've just got out of bed. You know the one: that time when the kids are possibly still asleep, the house is quiet and the hassles that might await you at work are still off in the distance. It's at this time that many people savour their most enjoyable cup of coffee of the entire day.

Why is that cup so enjoyable? Not just because it's likely to be enjoyed in peace, as you sit calmly and collect your thoughts for the day that awaits - there's more to it than that. Coffee does have a genuine calming effect that is capable of leaving you feel less light-headed on a morning, and here's how it works. When just the right amount of caffeine is added to your body, it slows down the supply of blood to your brain. It does so by tightening up blood vessels which are trying to rush blood to your brain when you first get up and out of bed. It's the reason you may feel a little light-headed, disoriented, or not quite yourself, until you've had a cup.

Now, a lovely cup of coffee is a huge part of my day (grande, extra hot, no foam latte, is how I specifically like it). And you know what? I often write my newspaper articles, blog posts or emails to clients, or do some of my most important work of the day with a fresh cup in hand, first thing in the morning – including the writing of this book. Yes - not a chapter of this book has been started without a fresh latte in hand as I sit down and prepare to write all this for you. It's true - if I can sit in my favourite coffee shop with a good book in one hand and a fresh latte made to my liking in the other, I find it to be one of the most positive and stimulating situations I can put myself in.

Something to make a note of: to make the most of any caffeine hit, try to pay attention to exactly when you want it to happen - and then enjoy it. Because it genuinely is a scientifically-proven stimulant that is going to make you feel nice and more alert – drunk in the right quantity. And what I mean by that is this: think about the second cup of coffee you might drink, later in the day, possibly after a stressful commute to work, having read and replied to a dozen unnecessary or unwelcome emails and had your first run-in with the boss or someone else at work who always seems to get your day off to a bad start. The caffeine hit second time round just isn't quite the same, is it?

And here's the other problem with excessive coffee: it's very easy to confuse exactly what it does for you. Sure, it will give you a slight boost or lift due to the caffeine and adrenaline it releases, the stuff that makes you feel alert and wanting to do things, but an excess of caffeine and the reverse is likely to happen. Too much too soon and you will drain your body of its adrenaline. With adrenaline drained from your body by an excess of caffeine, you're going to feel very tired, all the time.

Let me give you another example of how adrenaline works: what I've just described is the type of feeling that happens to runners involved in a big race – even a fun one such as the Great North Run. Participants are often so excited beforehand, just to be part of something so big and so good, that they are unable to keep emotions in check and will drain too much adrenaline. That means that 20 minutes or so into the race they're struggling to keep the pace and can't understand why they feel so exhausted, despite having done all of their training. Obviously, when they were in training, there was an absence of the pre-race excitement and all the adrenaline was kept in check, to be released slowly throughout the course of the training run, as and when it was needed.

Now think about the two o'clock lull that happens in every office, almost every day. You know the one - that time of the day when you're a little tired and wish you could perk yourself up a little to get you through the rest of the afternoon. Many people think a nice cup of coffee is just the stimulant they need to keep them alert when this happens. Yes, one cup is OK, but anything more than that and you will likely feel even more tired. And as you feel more tired, it's likely that you're in a self-perpetuating cycle. There's a constant temptation to keep downing the coffee thinking it's going to make you alert – when in reality, it's having the opposite effect and making you feel WORSE. You've only got so much adrenaline to be used each day, and pumping your body full with caffeine will make sure that your supply is emptied quickly.

Last thing on this: look around your office today, or even think about your own routine. How many cups of coffee are you drinking? If it's more than 2, maximum three, the effect that it's having may not be the one you're intending or imagining – and sure isn't a healthy one!

Is sitting the new smoking?

Here's a habit I KNOW you've got. Sitting is something that people once did only when they needed a rest – but, it seems, not any more. Sitting has now become what I call a 'dangerous norm', meaning everyone does it every day, so everyone thinks it's OK to keep doing it. Whether we're in your car, at work, out for dinner, having coffee, watching TV or using the computer, we're all constantly sitting.

Think about your typical daily routine for a moment, and you might realise that you spend an alarming number of hours in a chair. If it's more than 9, you could have a few unwanted (and unknown) health problems. Here's why.

Simply, we were not designed to sit. Our bodies are not shaped to do it, nor do they have the natural ability to cope with spending the whole time seated with pressure on the lower back and carrying the weight of the head as it drops forward when you sit. I'll happily bet that sitting has become so frequent and so extensive in your life that it's very unlikely you'll ever question how much of it you do. Everyone else is doing lots of it, so it must be OK, right? But here's something to consider: the health issues that occur as a result of this excess time spent sitting (such as bad backs, painful, swollen knees and tight, tense shoulder muscles) could be surfacing in our society YEARS later. As with the smoking habit of previous generations, nobody ever questioned it until studies of the health damage it did were produced and people started suffering, a few decades on.

The reality is this: you and I need to sit LESS. And here's a startling fact for you: Even just spending an hour in the sitting position, you reduce your body's ability to burn fat by up to 90% because it slows down your body's metabolism significantly. This can reduce the amount of good cholesterol in your body and without good cholesterol, you're at a greater risk of heart disease and diabetes.

Excess sitting in wrong positions (when you're slouched) is also the number one cause of back pain and neck and shoulder tension in the people who visit my physiotherapy clinic. And they're nearly always in their 40s and 50s. More: the excess pressure from poor sitting, when all of your body weight pushes down on your lower back and stresses joints, can lead to things like sciatica and cervical spondylitis (stiffness in neck joints), not to mention awkward looking postures. All of these things combined are the reasons why you shouldn't be surprised if your workplace introduces a standing desk area. I'm serious, too. They're really effective in allowing you to carry on with your work but reducing the impact through your spine significantly.

And while I'm on the subject of standing at work, let me tell you a true story.

How to exercise – even when you're at work

Now, I know that this section is all about unhealthy habits, but I want to show you an unusual way of turning an unhealthy habit into a VERY healthy habit. It's just going to require you to be open minded to the concept, and have an understanding of the benefits. What I'm going to share with you here is likely to benefit office workers who sit at a desk all day and parents (or grandparents) who are concerned about the amount of time their children spend sitting at a computer or playing video games.

Question: have you ever seen anyone who is at work running on a treadmill and still working on their computer? Picture that in your mind. A guy or woman in a suit, in a big office block, running or walking on a treadmill and taking a call or working on a laptop! Sounds farfetched? I saw this sort of thing happening regularly on a trip I once took to Boston when I was there attending a meeting. In the office space we were working from, the sight of people standing at desks and yes, exercising while working at laptops, could be seen all around me. And you know what? There was often a queue to get on that same treadmill, pretty much all day long.

I've already written many times about the dangers of sitting for extended periods. In the section above, I told you all about the long and short-term complications of spending too much time sitting, and said we all need to find ways to reduce the amount we do. One of those ways is to stand at work, or in your home office. After that trip to America, I talked this subject over with all my colleagues, and we came to the conclusion that we needed to start practising what we preach. So the standing desks are on order as I write this book. We're building part of my head office (on Raby Road in Hartlepool) into a standing room only area, and every member of staff is going to be spending at least 2-3 hours of their day in there. We're bringing in a soft-cushioned mat to stand on, to ease any pressure on knee and back joints, and we've talked through any modifications that might need to be made to footwear that staff currently wear, to make it more comfortable, safe and healthy to work in this new way.

Now, I did raise the possibility of a treadmill with a desk above it which would let my staff tap on a laptop or answer the phone at the same time as taking a gentle jog, but I got a few funny looks. So maybe I'll have to start with that in my own office and slowly but surely convince my staff of the health benefits of walking (or running) while working too.

On a serious note, standing desks and treadmills with desktops at work are becoming more common. Watch this space over the next few years as standing at work to answer the phone or use the computer becomes socially accepted. I bet that once YOU start to do it, you'll be left wondering why you didn't do it sooner. Aside from the obvious benefits like less back pain, a healthier-looking posture and more good cholesterol in your system, don't underestimate the extra energy and alertness you'll enjoy feeling from not being seated all day long.

If your kids or grandkids are always on the computer and you're worried about their posture, why not invest in a treadmill with a desk and tell them they can play on the computer to their hearts' content – as long as their little legs are working as fast as their fingers.

A few more tips to avoid prolonged sitting: next time you have a meeting, can you take a walk and do it ? If you need to talk for a while on your mobile phone, maybe go for a walk outside to do it so that you're walking, not sitting. And if you're meeting up with friends for a coffee this weekend, instead of sitting down to do it, find a nice park or beach and take a stroll with a take-away cup in hand (not too many though - remember caffeine is only helpful in small doses!)

The real reasons why TV is bad for your health

I've mentioned the dangers of sitting at work and playing video games, but I couldn't move on from this section without discussing the impact that sitting and watching TV simultaneously is likely to have upon your health – because it's rarely a good one.

The bad habit of watching too much TV nearly always gets worse in winter, when it's not uncommon to see a big change in people's health habits in general. You know how it goes in winter - you head home after work in the dark with nothing else on your mind other than to walk through the door, put the tea on, lock the front door for the night (knowing that nobody ever comes round when it's winter), then settle down on the couch for the evening and relentlessly flick through the TV channels to find something entertaining to watch to help pass the evening away until it's time to go to bed. All of this is usually done before 7pm and ensures another 3-4 hours sitting is added to the day. Add that to the time spent sitting during the day at work, and not forgetting the time spent sitting in the car during the daily commute, and winter represents a significant increase in the stress placed upon your body.

And you know what's really bad for your health, as well as spending too long sitting down to watch TV? It's the position most people have those TVs in. Or to be more precise, it's the position their head and neck is then going to be in, as a result. Let me explain: just about everybody has one of those big flat screen TVs these days. And don't they look great when you hang them on the wall? A big TV on the wall, high above a fire or mantelpiece, has almost become the centrepiece of most people's livings rooms these days and when you get back in after a long day at work, or just fancy a lazy day on the couch watching TV, then there's a good chance you're going to be spending hours looking at it – in a very unhealthy position.

You see, lots of people make the mistake of choosing what the TV looks like when it's in position over how healthy it is to have it there. You might not be aware of it, but having the TV above the level of your eyes if you're planning to watch it sitting on the couch, is a guaranteed way to increase neck, shoulder and eye problems. And probably one or two migraines and headaches along the way too.

How come? Well, it's all to do with your eyes having muscles and the fact that your eyes come with a natural downward tilt. It's the reason why when you stare down a corridor, 80% of what you see is the floor, and not the ceiling.

To help yourself understand this better, try this little exercise: lift your right arm up and hold it out straight in front of you. I'd guess that within 20-30 seconds your muscles would start to hurt, feel weak and then you'd feel a burning sensation. Next your arm will probably shake like mad and eventually you will have to drop it because it's so uncomfortable… did you try it?

When you have your TV above your natural eye line, you're asking the muscles in your eyes to do what you just tried doing with your arm. Queue a domino effect of problems starting with eye strain, neck pain because you tilt your head back to avoid the pain happening behind your eyes, and then comes a dose of shoulder pain as you try to limit the effect of holding your head in a position that's not familiar too you. All in all, it's not very healthy at all, and if you were to keep doing it, you'd have long term problems with all these areas.

Tip: There's a reason why TV stands are nearly all the same height and any decent one will always mean that if you're sitting on the couch watching TV, you'll be looking DOWN. Now, if you like to go to bed to watch TV, as I do, high up on the wall is the perfect place for it to be. Why? Well, now you know how your eyes work, think about what you see when you lie in bed – that's right, this time 80% of what you see is the upper part of the room and the ceiling. So it makes sense to have your TV higher up on the wall so that it's in line with your eyeline. When it comes to TV in the bedroom, the stand your telly comes with isn't an ideal choice – not if you like to lie back in bed with your head on a pillow. Do it this way and it should help you avoid migraines, headaches, eye trouble and muscle tension.

A lazy runner

Let's talk about another unhealthy habit – running! That's right, running. Let me explain to you why and how it becomes an unhealthy habit. It's not uncommon for people to get into the daily habit of going for a run, and doing so is great for heart and lungs. A quick run is perfect if you haven't got much time on your hands to do some exercise like swimming or cycling, which might take a little longer. However, there's a big but coming right up.

And here it is: one of the problems with enjoying going for a run or a gentle jog is that it's very easy to become lazy about doing it. Not lazy in the physical sense of avoiding effort, but in the routine you get into. Going for a run requires very little preparation or effort and it's over and done within 30 minutes or less (or at least it can be).

I call it the running trap, because running is just too convenient. Once you get into the habit of doing it, it's very difficult to get out of it. Running requires very little thought or planning. Finish work, head straight home and put your runners on and then out the door you go for a jog along the sea front, around the estate or the local park, or whichever route you've settled into. Within 30 minutes, your exercise for the day is done and dusted and the benefits felt. Shower included, it probably takes no more than 45 minutes to feel as healthy as you want to feel for the rest of the night.

Because of the amount of endorphins (the feel-good chemicals which are released during exercise) running daily can very easily become an addiction (not just a habit). But here's something to bear in mind that most people don't know: long-distance, cross-country style running is great for your body's strength and fitness, and even stamina, but it can have a negative effect on the flexibility of your joints and muscles. It can further restrict the natural flexibility that you're already losing on a daily basis, once you pass 40.

Let me tell you a painful story of a personal lesson I learned on this exact subject. A few years back I took some time out from playing cricket. Largely due to my commitments with working as a physio at a professional football club, I didn't have my weekends free to play cricket as I had nearly always done since I was about 13. And I'll be honest, in my teens and early twenties, it's safe to say I didn't always keep as fit as I do now. I'd label myself as a sprinter. In my school years and for a few after, I was able to run much more quickly over shorter distances than most, but I wasn't great at running more slowly for longer. So playing sports like cricket and football suited me and the quick bursts of speed I had helped me get between the wickets faster (when playing cricket) than most. Because of it, I'd always add a few extra runs to the score board that others might not have got. But when the physio career took off for me and I landed a job in professional football (meaning no time for cricket any more), I had to find something else to do to keep me fit and active.

So I started to jog, and bike ride. I very quickly realised that I loved to do both. Lots of reasons why, but I always felt that the 30 minutes or longer I had out on the road when I was running was my own. No one could get to me and I could be left alone to think, so I would always come back feeling clearer about my day or things that I needed to do. So I became addicted to running.

But then here's why happened next: when I quit my job in pro football to launch my private physio clinics, I went back to playing cricket. About seven years had passed since I'd played and I hadn't done much in the way of the sprinting (or running faster than jogging pace) that's needed when you play cricket. And 15 minutes into the second game of my first return season, I hit the ball, set off for what was to be a very quick run - and half way down the pitch felt the most intense pain in the back of my leg - I'd torn my hamstring. Painful? Oh yes! So much so that I could barely walk off the pitch.

Now, hamstring injuries often happen when you least expect them (by the way, the hamstring muscle is the one at the back of your thigh). And one of the things that makes you more likely to suffer a hamstring injury like I did on that day, is switching from a long period of time running at a slow steady pace to suddenly moving dynamically and explosively in training or games. I've even seen people suffer this type of injury after sprinting to get across the road to catch a bus!

Here's why it happened to me. Going for a run night after night shortened the length of my hamstrings (and all the other muscles, too). My muscles had become shorter, which meant that I was more likely to get injured as a result of it. The solution? Simple, I had to start doing more stretching of vital muscles - and start doing it daily. Hence how I found Yoga, and I can say for certain how beneficial it is in my life, and I'm still in my early 30s. It's something to bear in mind, and one of the reasons why it's really important for you to stretch daily - just 7 minutes on a morning is enough, and if you do it in the shower smothered in warm water, you're going to feel the benefits even more.

But here's another thing about running on pavements: have you ever thought about the impact that pounding the streets night after night is having upon your joints? If you're in your 50s and beyond, the last thing you need to be doing is adding to the wear and tear process that's already happening (aka arthritis). Even if you're wearing the best trainers, the stress you're putting on your knees and hips is beyond denial – and isn't good! What's worse, you're unlikely to notice until it's too late and the pain and swelling have arrived. Don't get me wrong, running is great for keeping things like your heart and lungs in good shape, but your knees and hips might have to pay the price in the long run if you're planning on doing it every night. And it's in the long run, perhaps in 10-15 years, where you'll find physical health problems that might stay with you for life.

It's true - every day my physio clinic is packed full of runners suffering with injuries like shin splints, IT band problems, tight Achilles muscles and even bad backs caused by too much running. So, here's what to do: find a balance somewhere between wanting to get fit (in the heart and lungs dept) and not doing your joints any harm in the long run (arthritis) because of it. Do your joints a big favour by considering other ways to keep fit and consider varying what you do. Even if the sun is shining after work and the running shoes are in the hallway when you walk through the door after a long day in the office, it pays to consider that going for yet another run may not be in the long term best interests of your health.

Here's a few suggestions to mix things up. Swimming might take a little longer to get done, but it's a great activity to increase your general all-round fitness. Maybe add in a bike ride once a week, even a session of yoga and/or Pilates. Doing this means that because you're having a couple of nights off from running, your joints are going to get a nice rest from the constant pounding it brings. Best of all, doing it this way, you're still working on your fitness and health in other ways, meaning your heart and lungs are getting the nice workout that will keep the doctor happy and you feeling great.

If you really can't cut down on the running night after night, consider doing part of your run on grass or sand, as just changing the surface you run on will make all the difference – even more so in a few years' time - to the inevitable aches and pains in your joints that await if you don't.

Chapter Eight

They laughed when I paid a private physio, but when they saw me walking again...

. . . .

When word spread in my industry that I'd been asked to publish a book like this, I was asked by my peers, and even one of two of my competitors, to include a few sections on physio, and specifically to write a few words that would set the record straight on what it is, what it does and who it can help. You see, there's lots of confusion about physio out there in society – made worse by many private physios who operate what I call 'after-work clinics', where they have day jobs and show up when it's convenient for them with no real commitment to their clients or patients. The freely-available government-funded physio service is moving faster towards a fully hands-off approach, which is confusing and disappointing for patients and leaves many wondering why they went to see a physiotherapist and came back with only a few scraps of general advice and some sheets of exercises to work on at home. Besides, what sort of advocate for my profession would I be if I didn't include a section on physiotherapy in a book about healthy habits?

Setting the record straight about physiotherapy

So hereafter I'm going to set the record straight and show you how going to see a good private physio might be a valuable habit to add to your life.

It's true - physio is one of the best ways to keep active and healthy, particularly if you're over 50, and it's a great way to avoid having to take painkillers or bothering the GP for things like back, knee, neck and shoulder pain.

I'm going to give you a back-stage tour and take you behind the scenes of what physiotherapy really is and does - and more to the point, I'm going to show you why it might be able to help you. I'm about to share with you one or two interesting stories about physio. I'll show you who it's really for (it might shock you) and tell you how to make sure you get the best out of seeing a physio, should you decide to do so. I'll leave you with some tips on how to pick a good one, as well as clearing up a few dangerous half-truths and myths that exist about physio. These wrong ideas can stop people from getting access to the type of A-grade advice and physical treatment that could well be the critical missing link in their goal of staying active and healthy long into their 50s, 60s and beyond.

First, let me tell you about one of my favourite stories from inside my physio room. It's about a lady who once came to see me with nagging shoulder pain and almost did something that she most certainly would have later come to regret.

So there I was in my treatment room one day in my clinic in Hartlepool when in walked this very pleasant young lady who had been advised to see me by a colleague of hers. He had told her I'd be the right person to look at her tight, tense and painful shoulder muscle and put it right. Nothing out of the ordinary so far.

But then what happened was this. Vicki, the lady in question, had never had physio in the past, so she wasn't sure exactly what would happen or how her session with me would work. And because she was a little unsure about what was going to happen inside the treatment room, she started to ask me a series of questions. One of them was this:

"Do I have to take my clothes off, Paul?"

She was understandably nervous about this new physio experience she was going through, and asking many questions in an attempt to find reassurance as to what was going to happen next. So she wasn't really listening to any of the answers I was giving. And when I answered with a NO, she didn't hear me. As she asked me this question, I was walking towards the door of my physio room, about to nip out to replace a bottle of massage oil. This would also give Vicki time to get settled, take her shoes and jacket off and get comfortable on the massage bed before I went to work on relaxing her tight shoulder muscles, which had been caused by poor sitting posture at work.

So, even though I had told her not to take her clothes off, she proceeded to do so. Luckily I walked back into the room just in time to stop her from going through with it. She might have regretted it if she had done so. Let me explain why. Taking your clothes off in front of a medical professional is one thing, but taking them off in front of your future boss - well that's another story altogether. You see Vicki is now the person who runs my office!

Yes - not long after that same physio session with me I offered her the very first full-time job I had ever given out. I guess you could say the laughs and the fun we had as a result of that almost so-embarrassing situation in my treatment room told me that Vicki had just the type of fun personality I wanted in my growing physio business. So when she returned to the clinic a few days later I offered her a job, and she accepted.

Since that day, we've joked about it with other clients

of my clinic on many occasions. And they love it – it puts them right at ease and I think it does so because there are lots of questions people wish they had answers too before going to see a physio, and 'do I have to take my clothes off?' is just one of them.

We decided to put the whole funny story onto a video and share it with all the clients who book appointments at my clinic. It clears up a lot of confusion about what happens inside the treatment rooms of a physiotherapy clinic, and I know for sure that many of my clients are very happy when we show it to them. In the video, Vicki and two other members of my staff (one of whom also began as a client/patient of mine before taking a job with my clinic) talk about all the things they were thinking before they came for their first physio session with me, what they thought about it immediately after, and what they now know about how physio really works and who it helps, since they have experienced it from both sides of the treatment room door.

The video of Vicki describing that day when she almost took her clothes off has been watched thousands of times now. It's a very entertaining video that puts our patients and ease before they arrive – it makes them laugh too. If you'd like to see it for yourself, or you're thinking about going to see a physio anytime soon and you would just like to get a REAL insight as to what is going to happen when you get there, then you can watch the full video (11 minutes 19 seconds) on YouTube. Search for the 'Paul Gough Physio' channel and the video is titled, 'Do I Have To Take My Clothes Off? Physio FAQs'. Watch the video and you'll get honest and emotive answers to the most common questions people ask before going to see a physio, from three ladies who have all been in that same situation – if you are ever thinking of going to see a physio, you'll be glad you watched it. Anyhow, I hope you enjoy it! Now let's move on and talk about this…

A physio clinic up three steep flights of stairs

The waiting room of one of the busiest chiropractic and physio clinics in central London is at the top of three very steep flights of stairs. Add the fact that this same clinic lacks any form of nearby car parking and you'd be forgiven for thinking that such a building would be the worst kind to house the cure for anyone suffering with back, knee or ankle pain (or any type of physical pain which would make climbing stairs difficult).

Take a minute to digest what I just wrote, and picture a clinic for people with painfully bad backs, on the third floor, with steep stairs and no lift. How would you ever even manage to get there if you couldn't park your car? It could be a long walk if you've got back pain. But it's there, it's very popular and here's why. This particular clinic is for people who refuse to let their back or knee pain get so bad that it stops them from getting up stairs. On my first trip to this clinic to meet the guy who owns it, I was delighted at how busy his clinic was, but shocked at the lack of accessibility and the slightly awkward location. Three flights of stairs is a long way for anyone to have to climb, but for a person suffering with back pain - surely no one would ever go there?

The doctor who owns the clinic is named Mikael. And here's what he told me:

'Ground floor physio or chiropractor premises are not needed in London because people come to see us well before they're actually in any pain. Floor 3 works well because the people down here understand the true value and the real reason you should go and see someone like a physio.'

Take note of this, particularly if you're trying your best to keep as active and healthy as you can for the next few decades of your life. You see, some people, particularly in the North East where I'm from, make the mistake of thinking that physios and chiropractors are only needed in emergency situations, such as when you're in severe back or knee pain, or whatever it is that might be hurting. But Mikael is suggesting that people who go to his medical facility see it from a different angle. They never let problems such as back pain get so severe that they're unable to climb stairs.

Think of it like this: you're unlikely to go to the dentist only when your teeth are hurting. Sure, there will be times in your life when you'll have to do that, but as a general rule, you see your dentist every six months, even if you're not in pain or discomfort. And I think that's how people should start to see physio. It's OK to turn up when you're in a lot of pain because yes, you're going to get the relief you're looking for. But why wait until it gets bad? Wouldn't it be better to get things like your back and knees checked regularly in the same way as your teeth? After all, what's more important? I know living without my teeth wouldn't be ideal, but I could easily get some false ones and still go on eating what I wanted. How do you replace a severely damaged spine? And sure, they can replace a knee these days, but the operation is quite an ordeal, and it's never the same afterwards. So if you're thinking physio is only for people in pain, I'd encourage you to think differently. Some of the healthiest and most active people I know go to see a physio to ensure they stay that way, not to get back to living that way.

7 reasons why seeing a physio is better than taking painkillers

I'm about to show off one of the biggest reasons why so many people love coming to rely on a hands-on physio – and that's quite simply because it's the polar opposite to relying upon painkillers. Because I want you to understand how much value a physio can bring to your lifestyle, I want you to take a quick look at 5 reasons why physio can often be a better option that taking painkillers.

1) No nasty lasting side effects.

2) It wins the war - and NOT just the little battles. Physio gets to the very root of your pain to stop it, not mask it with little victories that don't last or mean anything in the end.

3) You're not reliant on physio for months or years.

4) Physio doesn't lure you into telling yourself 'I'm doing OK today' to be hit hard by pain when you didn't expect it.

5) The effects of physio don't wear off after just four hours.

Now don't get me wrong - taken at the right time, and for the right reasons, I encourage anyone to take painkillers, IF the GP advises it. But I disagree wholeheartedly with painkillers being prescribed without the root cause of the problem being addressed first. If that isn't done, your problem WILL come back, and it will lead to a dependency on painkillers (instant gratification). This is how people get hooked on them for years and end up with the side effects I mentioned above.

Many people I help think of physio as an escape route from relying upon painkillers and prescriptions, and it's true. Physio lets you get active and healthy again on your terms, at a convenient time, without any fear of side effects or addiction.

How to pick the right physio (for you)

So maybe I've got you thinking that going to see a physio the next time your back, knee, neck or shoulder is playing up is a good idea? If so, I want you to know how to pick a good one when you need to. So with that in mind, here are 7 questions that any good physio should be able to answer.

1) Ask the physio if they use their hands. This is important, because if you're wanting relief from things like joint pain and muscle tension, there's no better way to achieve it than by using expert techniques such as massage, PNF stretching and joint realignment, which must be done by hand. My clients are assured that at least 85% of their time with me will be hands-on. Anything less and I wouldn't be offering them value for their money.

2) Ask if the physio has another job. A big problem in the physio industry is that many private physios have other jobs. Most still work for the NHS through the day and I'm sorry to say that as a result they may not be 100% committed to their private clients. Besides, if you choose an NHS physio who moonlights and does a little after-hours private physio, all you're going to get is what you would have got over in the free system – which is unlikely to be the hands-on physical-style therapy you want and need.

3) They must be CSP, HPC and BUPA registered. The reason why these three registrations are so important is that the physio will have had to go through many checks to get registered. The CSP and HPC are pretty standard in terms of safety and credibility, confirming that the physio is who they say they are and is as qualified as you hope, but the BUPA accreditation is much more difficult to achieve. BUPA is relentless when it comes to checking that your work is up to standard, clinic premises are up to scratch, all your liability, medical and professional insurance is up to date and that your care plans and treatment interventions are solid. So, HPC and CSP are the bare minimum requirement, but if you're looking for the gold seal of approval, BUPA recognition is a good one to ask for.

4) Own premises. Many part-time physios just rent a room at the back of a GP premises or a sports centre, or somewhere like that. And that's fine. It's just not great. It's also a good indicator that the physio is just doing it for a bit of extra cash (harsh but true). Renting rooms in sports centres is where I started out, but I did it with the full intention of getting out and into my own place to give my clients a better experience as quickly as possible.

5) Full-time secretary. If you ring a physio during the day and no one answers the phone, it's a good sign that it's a one-man band operation. Again, that's fine, but it's not great. The real success of my clinic has been in finding the most helpful, warm and friendly secretaries that I could hire to give a warm greeting to any potential new client who shows an interest in coming to see me.

6) Price and availability. If you're calling a good physio, you'll struggle to get an appointment immediately and you should be paying at least £55-65 per visit for a half hour session - great hands-on physios are hard to come by because they are so popular. The best indicator you can find is the 'how soon' test. If you ring at 9 am and they invite you to come down for 10 am, chances are they are not in great demand, so perhaps they're not the kind of physio you want to go and see.

As for the investment in going to see a good private physio, the best physios can command a fee of anything from £55 - £65 (higher in London) for each visit, although results-orientated physios will offer packages and programmes that are guaranteed to work. Expect to pay slightly more for the first session (initial consultation) because it's the most valuable and it's where the really clever and important work is done by the physio - figuring out what's gone wrong, and what to do about it.

7) Ask what they specialise in. If the physio can't answer it in an instant or you get a muffled or stifled answer, perhaps one that includes a long list of injuries, then the chances are that this physio doesn't have a speciality, or doesn't know the answer. And that's fine. It's just not great. Because if they don't know themselves what they specialise in, how can they route all their training and efforts towards becoming even better at it? They can't. This means you're not going to get the specialist help you need. And that's a problem for the physio industry, as many physios don't know what they're good at or what they want to be good at, or even who they want to help.

So there you have it. To wrap up this section on physiotherapy, those are my 7 ways to cherry-pick the perfect physio, one who is going to be an ally in your attempt to keep active and healthy in your 50s, 60s and beyond.

OK, let's move on and talk about some ways to keep you *out of a physio room in the first place.*

Chapter Nine

Fatal health mistakes

(and top tips to stop the most common issues)

■■■■■■■■■■■■■■■

If you and I were introduced to each other by a mutual friend, I bet that as soon as you realised I was a physiotherapist, the first question you'd ask me would go something like this:

'Oh, you're a physio are you? Whilst you're here, can I just ask you a quick question - what's the best thing to do for my bad back (or knee or shoulder etc)?'

It happens nearly everywhere I go. And it's really nice, to be honest. I never get tired of being able to help people and it's often just a simple case of *do this, but don't do that!* My first response to that type of question is often NOT to tell the person asking what to do, but to tell them what NOT to do. You see, simply eliminating the things that make problems worse usually makes a significant difference before someone like me even has to go and do anything by hand in the physio room.

So with that in mind, this next chapter is devoted to highlighting what NOT to do to make things naturally better.

Let's start with...

6 things to avoid if you want a speedy end to back pain

1) Rest - too much of it can often mean you're making your back WEAKER and therefore more prone to problems further down the line – and definitely this is true the older your body gets. It's because muscles in your body get stronger as you move. You're designed to be active and as they say, *if you don't use it, you lose it.* It's that simple! Yet because you're feeling some form of discomfort or stiffness, you're tempted to rest up for a little while and just wait for it to go away. Problem is, some people forget to get going again, and years later when they go to see a physio the problem is much more difficult to solve than the initial pain they started out with.

2) Do not rely solely on painkillers. Doing that means you'll never get to the root cause of your back pain in the first place. Most people agree that painkillers aren't the best option. In the right situation, during the first few days of back pain, I think it's fine to take the right ones. But only if some sustainable solution is being prescribed at the same time – like physio.

3) Doing the wrong exercises at the wrong time. I see this all the time. Most people I meet with back pain say they've tried exercises before they arrive for treatment. Usually they've made their problems worse because they've been doing the wrong exercises, for the wrong reasons. In my experience, exercises do very little to ease back pain. They do, however, make it less likely to come back (big difference). But that's something that most people don't get. It's best not to do exercises when you're in pain, as you're only going to make things worse. Get hands on physio and posture advice first, then begin the exercises to make your body stronger and make you less likely to suffer again, any time soon.

My tip for exercises that make back pain less likely – use Pilates-style ones to give your muscles some much-needed control, mixed with a touch of yoga to make your back more flexible.

4) Avoid living with a neoprene back support. Wearing one of these every day will weaken the muscles around your lower back, so that within three months, maybe less, your lower back is going to be in a worse state than it was before you started wearing one. It's very similar to resting for too long. Sure, it feels nice when you start to wear it, and that's the problem. It's so easy to be lured into a false sense of security because of the drop in back pain, but if you're not careful, you can end up on a self-perpetuating cycle until you're a *bona fide* member of the life-long back pain club. And trust me.... there are much better clubs to join than that one. The members are all wishing they knew how to get out of it!

5) Sitting for long periods. 9 out of 10 back problems are made worse by sitting. I've mentioned this a few times in this book now, but let me point it out again. Think about how much time we now spend sitting and it's not difficult to work out why so many people aged 50+ are struggling with back pain. Try to cut this out and you'll see a gradual drop in back pain.

Here's a simple trick that I use myself to reduce the amount of sitting I do. Next time your phone rings or you know you're going to be on the phone for a while - **take a walk while you're doing it.** It's great for mental stimulation as well as your heart and lungs and takes some pressure off your lower back. Whatever you're chatting about on the phone, you will sound much more positive – you'll leave the person you're talking to wondering why you've got so much energy and enthusiasm in your voice.

6) Avoid wearing the wrong footwear. If you're wearing sandals, high heels or plimsoll-style trainers, you're adding massive amounts of stress to your lower back and increasing the length of time you will suffer. High heels are lethal – there's unlikely to be anything you could wear on your feet that is going to add to back pain as high heels do. Why? Well, there's no cushioning to absorb shock or impact from the hard pavement, so your knees and hips (and eventually your lower back) get damaged by the constant pounding every time you walk. Sure, they might look nice with the right dress, but you'll pay the price later with a bad back, not to mention an Achilles tendon that is likely to be very painful and tight the day you stop wearing them.

Plimsolls and sandals have a similar effect – they might look nice and feel comfortable when you wear them causally in summer, but because your foot is able to move around freely inside them, this adds stress and pressure to your lower back muscles. It's OK at first, but over time it's going to accumulate and you're going to suffer.

So there you have it - the top 6 things I recommend you take note of, look out for and ultimately stop doing completely, if you want to ease back pain, or lower the risk of ever suffering from it. Because the chances are that one day you will. More than 20 million people in Britain suffer from it every day, and at least 8 out of 10 people will at some point have their enjoyment of life interrupted by it.

That said, let me answer this next common question...

Why does back pain happen anyway?

Sometimes it happens. You're chugging along nicely. You feel fit and well and think your health problems are way off in the future, something to worry about another day. Then suddenly, you feel something's not quite right with your lower back. Maybe you even begin to kid yourself that it's nothing, that it will go away on its own. Or you pass it off as having just slept awkwardly, or something simple like that. But there's no obvious reason why. No clue. No real explanation. And when it happens, it leaves you suffering with back pain for much longer than you should.

So let's look at some common reasons why back pain happens, so that you can look out for them and know to act instantly to get your back looked at properly, if you think any of them has happened to you.

1) It could be a simple case of your lower back muscles finally packing up after years of overuse.

2) Maybe you suffered some back pain years ago and thought nothing of it at the time, but the real damage has been building slowly ever since and it's finally decided to surface now that your body isn't quite as flexible or as strong as it once was.

3) Perhaps you sit a lot? Maybe you sit at work or in your car, or maybe you've just picked up a bit of a bad habit that means you slouch when you're watching TV, or maybe you sleep in a funny way, such as on your front?

4) Maybe you're the one person in the house that is left to do all the housework, who is always cleaning the floor and picking things up after the kids or grandkids, or you spend time in the garden attending to its needs and constantly stressing your back whilst doing it? If so, then the toll all this has taken over the years is perhaps finally beginning to surface in the form of the back pain and stiffness you're now suffering.

And so the list goes on. Rarely does the reason for back pain, or the root cause of it, ever get more complex than anything you've just read above. In fact, I often argue that back pain is inevitable, that it's actually the sign of an active and on-the-go lifestyle where you've put to good use everything you've been given. It's just a shame that when you hit 40, definitely 50, and most certainly 60, that the really strong lower back you had when you were younger isn't the same any more. However, it's often nothing that can't be helped if you get it looked at quickly and follow one or two bits of advice.

The stats show that at least 8 out of 10 people will suffer with a bad back. And here's something that all of those people should have been told: chances are, if you've suffered back pain lasting for longer than 9 days, **it isn't likely to go away on its own**. That means you must do something about it - something that involves more than just rest or taking painkillers.

If back pain ever happens to you, here are a few suggestions.

Insider tips to reduce back pain

So now you know what causes back pain and how to stop it getting worse, and you're beginning to turn yourself into an expert, I want to add to the value you're getting from reading this book by showing you what you can do to ease back pain should it occur, as well as lower the risk that it will ever happen to you.

1. Avoid sitting cross-legged

Your spine isn't designed to twist or turn. Sitting in a cross-legged position is contributing to back pain because of that little-known fact.

2. Sleep with a pillow between your knees

It might be difficult at first, but if you can persist, it lowers the amount of rotation/twisting happening at your spine during the night. If you sleep on your side, a pillow between your legs will keep your spine in a nice position and this will reduce tension at your lower back - meaning you're likely to wake up in the morning in less pain and able to move more freely.

3. Avoid sleeping on your stomach

There is no faster way to do self-inflicted damage to your spine and lower back than by sleeping on your stomach. Avoid this position at all costs.

4. Change your mattress every 5 years

I get asked 'should I change my mattress?' just about every day. It's almost impossible to answer, as everyone has a different response to changing a mattress or the type they sleep on. What I can say is this: if you haven't changed your mattress in the last five years, then it's about time you did. You're unlikely to be getting the support for your lower back that you really need.

5. Get physical with physiotherapy

There isn't a faster way to end back pain than by going to see a physio. Getting to see a *hands-on* specialist physiotherapist means you're going to get very fast access to care that will soothe and relax those tight, aching lower back muscles, loosen and lubricate stiff, stuck and painful joints, and strengthen your body so you can go back to doing the things you love.

You can often leave a good physio with concerns eased and physical pain reduced inside 30-40 minutes.

6. Daily lower back exercise rituals – yoga and Pilates

If you can get into the routine or good habit of doing simple stretches and strengthening of your lower back muscles, you will benefit right through your 50s, 60s and beyond. In the same way as you brush your teeth twice a day to keep them clean and avoid pain, you need to look at working on your back in a similar way.

7. Stay hydrated

This is a BIG office worker mistake that could be zapping your energy and increasing lower backache. One really simple way to avoid it is to cut out the stuff that makes you dehydrated in the first place, things like excessive coffee, tea, alcohol and energy drinks. You'll be dehydrated if you drink too much of them and more likely to suffer from back pain.

So there you have it. Why back pain happens anyway, how to avoid back pain and what to do about back pain. You're now definitely becoming an expert on this topic!

For more back pain tips like this, please visit www.paulgoughphysio.com/back-pain, where there is a 12-page special report (currently free) waiting for you. It will give you instant access to the best ways to end back pain without taking painkillers or bothering the GP, and could reduce the risk of surgery.

Why it pays to know more about your knees

The reality is that like back pain, some kind of knee pain happens to just about everyone over the age of 50. What most people don't know is that the two go hand in hand. It's true - if your knees are not healthy, the chances are you'll also pay a price with back pain. And vice versa. It's all to do with the way you walk or sit to avoid pain in one or the other.

So let's look at what you can do to limit knee pain.

Most of the knee pain you're likely to suffer in your 50s and beyond is caused by a process simply called 'wear and tear of the joint surfaces'. Some GPs call it degeneration, or if they're going to be precise, they might use the term 'osteoarthritis'. Want to know what I call it? An inevitable consequence of active and healthy living. And there's not much you can do to stop it. Sure, you can slow it down and limit the effects, but wear and tear of joint surfaces is inevitable for someone who's been active for five or six decades.

But please don't let anyone tell you there is nothing you can do to stop knee pain – there ARE things you can do about it, most of the time. It's just that as you've lived your life, gone about your day and walked here to there, run, cycled, even just done your shopping or looked after the kids, over the years they've all added stress to the surface of your knee. And the nice soft cartilage you had in your 20s and 30s to protect your knee joints isn't as soft as it was by the time you reach 50. Think of a new surface being laid on a road. At first it's very soft and smooth to drive over, but day after day, week after week, because of the excess pressure put on it by the cars which drive over it, not forgetting changes in temperature, that same road surface within a few years will be riddled with cracks and potholes that make driving very uncomfortable. And it's the same with your knee. Those same cracks and potholes are happening inside your knee joint, and that's what causes the noises you might hear – it's just the two surfaces grinding together. That's why your knee joint can so easily become painful and stiff, not to mention swollen.

A quick note on swelling. If it happens to you, it's a sure-fire sign that the surface of your knee is beginning to wear away, and/or that one of the ligaments has been damaged. If your knee is swollen, it's going to help you to know that your problem isn't the swelling itself. No, you need to find out what has CAUSED the swelling. So if you're ever making a trip to a GP because your knee is swollen, you need to leave knowing why. Sounds so simple, but believe me I have heard from so many people who go to see their GP and leave having been told that they have a problem with swelling of the knee. They don't, they have a cartilage (or ligament) problem, and that's causing the swelling. And unless you get to the bottom of it and find a solution, it's guaranteed to come back. With that in mind. here are...

Secret tips to ease knee pain

As with easing and ending back pain, there are things you can be doing to ease knee pain naturally - that means without taking painkillers or needing injections or surgery.

First, make sure your knee muscles are strong enough to cope with the life you want to live. These days, everyone thinks the answer to any problem or physical pain is to just 'do some exercises'. As if any will do. Yes, doing exercises is <u>one</u> of the secrets to ending and easing knee pain naturally. But there's a right way and a wrong way to go about it.

And here's the right way: If your knee is painful or swollen, the first thing you have to do is STOP exercising. If it's not too bad, you can do a little bit of something like swimming (but not breast stroke) and take a gentle walk for 20 minutes or so on the flat, but you should not be carrying on with your usual routine, because you'll only make things worse. A knee joint that's painful and swollen is a sign that your knee isn't strong enough. It can happen for any reason, even no reason at all, but you need to understand there's a HUGE difference between *exercising* and *doing exercises*. The latter is what you need to recover a knee joint that hurts.

My tip: focus on improving the strength and control of your quad muscles. They're the big powerful muscles at the front of your knee and the more support you can get from them, the less pain you'll notice at the knee. Having strong quad muscles lowers your wear and tear risk too. But you also need to consider having lower back muscles that are strong and hips that move freely. You need to be wearing the right footwear with enough cushion to absorb shock (the shock you get every time your foot lands when you walk) and be sure your feet are in the right position in those shoes you're wearing, too.

For that to happen effortlessly, consider wearing specially-made foot orthotics (inserts). They really help people who are suffering from the state of their knees, or anyone who is just concerned about the overall health of their knees. More: if you like to be especially active, then wearing foot orthotics which slip inside your shoes and help keep your body in the right position is likely to make a significant and positive difference to how your knees feel and how healthy you're able to keep.

OK, that's your lower back and knees taken care of – now let's move higher up your body and talk about what to do to stop unwanted neck and shoulder pain.

For more knee pain tips like this, please visit this special information website:

www.paulgoughphysio.com/knee-pain. You'll find a free 13-page report waiting for you which shows you even more great ways to end knee pain without taking painkillers, injections or bothering the GP. It could even reduce the risk of surgery.

Why neck or shoulder pain is often an annoying daily nag

One of the greatest mysteries of being 50+ is the sudden onset of shoulder tension and general neck stiffness. It often creeps up on people with zero warning and usually offers no explanation as to why you might all of a sudden wake up one morning with the type of neck pain that is daily, annoying and nagging – to the point where it can make it very difficult to enjoy life.

It often happens due to an accumulation of things, such as sleeping with two pillows (instead of one), reading in bed, spending all day looking at a desk or computer screen, cleaning the house, ironing, preparing family meals and even reading the newspaper first thing in the morning.

Now, you might think all of those things I've just mentioned are fairly simple, even trivial things that shouldn't really cause neck or shoulder pain. And you'd be right. But like anything which is done repetitively, no matter how small a task, eventually the impact accumulates, to surface a few years later in the form of pain, stiffness and tension.

Let's look at reading before bed - who doesn't love to read before they go to bed? It's likely to be a habit you've had since your mother or father started to read to you before bed when you were a child. It's something you've no doubt done for your own children and will continue to do for any grandchildren you may have. But think about the position your head is in when you're reading. It's likely to be always looking DOWN.

Now, what most people don't know about the head is that it's designed to be in a position where *your ears are vertically in line with your shoulders*. As soon as you begin to look down (such as when you're reading a book), those ears are not in line any more. Again, that's OK if you only do it occasionally. But if you're doing it every day, it's going to cause you a problem and after a few years, your head will end up in a position that's out of line. If the habit continues when you're driving, watching TV, sitting at a desk or in the kitchen when cooking tea, or looking down to do the ironing for an hour or more a few times per week, it's easy to see why your ears may not be level with your shoulders by the time you reach 50! To be honest, these days, it's rare that I see teenagers with their heads in the right position. I can only shudder to think what their posture will look like in 30 to 40 years from now.

But there's another problem with reading before bed, and it's the reason why lots of people end up with tight shoulder muscles and a very stiff neck, and even suffer from tension-type headaches throughout the night and first thing in the morning. When you're reading that book, you have to hold it in place to keep reading it. And that means you're tensing your muscles, because holding the book in place is going to put your neck into a locked and rigid position. Again, it's not too bad at first, but doing it night after night isn't helpful. My tip: if you enjoy reading before bed, try not to do it for any longer than for 20 minutes (or at least change position if you do).

And here's one more thing about this - the number of pillows you sleep with can also affect the position of your head and therefore the amount of pain you will suffer. Think about it for a minute. If you sleep with two thick or heavy pillows, it is going to push your head forward, so those ears are not in line with your shoulders again. Not a problem at first, but 10 years on, after spending 8 hours per night sleeping like that, it's guaranteed to leave you with a less than healthy posture. I nearly always recommend one thin pillow over two every time (unless you have a specific neck condition which requires more). And yes, it will feel awkward at first, but after about two weeks or so, your body will get used to its new sleeping position and you will see and feel a remarkable improvement in the tension you *won't* be feeling in your neck and shoulders.

I know these are tiny little changes that I'm offering up to you, but believe me, in the same way that lots of tiny little things add up to cause problems in your 50s and 60s, lots of tiny little improvements or alterations will also combine to leave you feeling less stiff, less tense and living with more energy and freedom than anyone else you know. Would that be nice? Thought so!

Now let me finish by saying this: from what you've just read in these last few sections, and I'm hoping you'll agree, the most valuable part of getting access to a specialist physio like me, or any other health care professional for that matter, isn't necessarily to get the hands-on treatment (although that's VERY important). No, going to see a specialist physio is worth it - just to get the *'do this, but don't do that'* advice that will provide you with clarity and hope for a future that can be free from things like back, knee and neck pain.

Your investment in going to see a specialist physio will mean an end to confusion, solid answers to questions that concern you, an accurate 'what's gone wrong' (the diagnosis) and an expected timeframe for a full recovery that is safe and will mean less problems in the future.

I couldn't finish this book without reminding you that *physiotherapy is a perfect solution for anyone who enjoys their health too much to ever risk losing it.* From my own experience, what I've found from being a physio and why most people choose to come and see me, is this: **Most**

of the time, most people are able to live with the pain that they are suffering - they just don't want to. Don't wait for the pain to be so severe that you feel you have a justification to go and see one – that's not how you'll get the best from what someone like me does to improve health.

For more neck and shoulder pain tips like this, please visit this special information website: www.paulgoughphysio.com/neck-shoulder-pain where you'll find waiting for you a currently free 14-page special report which shows you even more of the best ways to end shoulder pain before it causes severe headaches and disturbs sleep.

Chapter Ten

The death of good health habits

....

I'm nearly done writing this book for you now. But before I wrap it up, I just want to point one final thing out. And it's this: **the death of any good health habit is TIME.**

Too often I meet people who told me that 6 months ago (sometimes as long as a year, even 5, 10 and 20 years ago), they wanted to do something to turn around their failing health and get started with something like physio or better exercise habits or change their lifestyle choices for the better. But for one reason or another, they didn't get round to it. It's as if they fully understand, even know for sure, that there would be a benefit to the changes they were planning to make, but they just couldn't go that final step and actually do it. And at the end of the day, nothing happens until someone takes some action.

My challenge to you is to take action on some of the

things you've learned in this book, NOW. Like RIGHT NOW! I really hope you will. Find just one thing in this book that you liked the sound of, commit to doing it and **don't stop**. It could be anything from changing how much coffee you drink during the day to when you eat or read, or simply changing the route or the shoes you wear when you exercise to protect vital joints. All the tips I've revealed in this book will make a difference to any person's health - and that most definitely includes YOU. Once you've made one improvement to your life and you start to enjoy the benefits, go ahead and make another, and another and another. And just keep going. Imagine if you made one improvement each month - one year from now there'll be 12 healthier things happening in your life that you're not currently doing – and that has to look and feel good, right?

This doesn't have to be the end...

Each week I talk directly to about 100,000 people about ways to improve their health, either through my weekly health and fitness columns in the *Northern Echo* and *Hartlepool Mail*, or via email. More than 20,000 people (at the time of publishing this book) from around the world have joined my health tips email list and are now enjoying receiving regular health advice from me delivered directly to their inbox.

I firmly believe they signed up for my emails because

each one understands that while it's easy to be inspired to go and do good things after reading a thoughtful book like this, when becoming healthier is top of your mind, it doesn't last. Inspiration wears off! And if you're not getting a continuous stream of good and positive advice fed to you on a regular basis, then you will likely fall back into the old unhealthy routines.

So, a good thing for you to do next would be to visit my website and leave your name and email address - then I'll know to send you more health tips like the ones you've enjoyed reading in this book. Here's where to do that: www.paulgoughphysio.com/gifts

Special bonus: healthy gifts and goodies for you

And when you do type this web address into Google www.paulgoughphysio.com/gifts, just fill out the quick form on the screen, and I'll send you some other information to help keep you healthy, active and mobile... including my **10-Day Healthy Meal Planner** loaded with recipes for all the family (value £33) as well as my **7 Day, 7 Minute Stretching Routine Guide,** which is perfect for any person aged 50 or over who wishes they were a bit more flexible and supple (value £27). You'll be able to see them both instantly when you enter your name and email address at www.paulgoughphysio.com/gifts

If you follow the simple instructions in both the healthy resource manuals I'm going to give you, you will notice a positive difference to how healthy you look and feel. Make sure you get them all (and I guarantee there will be more healthy gifts like this given out over the coming months and years when you join my email list).

So please go here now: www.paulgoughphysio.com/gifts

Your healthy resource library

. . . .

If you would like more in-depth information and self-help tips on any of the common topics you see listed below, then please just visit the web address printed next to each. When you get there, you'll see a special tips report I have prepared for you and more information on ways to get the help you need.

Back pain: www.paulgoughphysio.com/back-pain

Neck or shoulder pain:
www.paulgoughphysio.com/neck-shoulder-pain

Sports injury recovery tips:
www.paulgoughphysio.com/sports-injury-clinic

Knee pain: www.paulgoughphysio.com/knee-pain

Foot and ankle pain:
www.paulgoughphysio.com/foot-ankle-pain

Postnatal back pain recovery:
www.paulgoughphysio.com/postnatal-back-pain

51 FAQ's of physiotherapy: www.paulgoughphysio.com

Talk to a physio from the comfort of your own home

More, if you feel as though speaking to a specialist about any health-related problem you're currently having, then I can also offer you a free 20-minute telephone consultation with a physiotherapist from my own clinic.

You can do that by visiting www.paulgoughphsio.com/talk and leaving your details or by calling my clinic directly using Freephone: 0800 043 8671. Please tell the person answering the phone that you have been reading this book and wish to take advantage of the generous offer to speak with a physio for free, and you will be taken care of from there.

Health Disclaimer

We make every effort to ensure that we accurately represent the injury advice and prognosis displayed throughout this book. However, examples of injuries and their prognosis are based on typical representations of those injuries that we commonly see in our physiotherapy clinics. The information given is not intended to apply to every individual's potential injury. As with any injury, each person's symptoms can vary widely and each person's recovery from injury can also vary depending upon background, genetics, previous medical history, application of exercises, posture, motivation to follow physio advice and various other physical factors.

It is impossible to give a 100% complete accurate diagnosis and prognosis without a thorough physical examination, and likewise the advice given for management of an injury cannot be deemed fully accurate in the absence of this examination from one of the Chartered Physiotherapists at Paul Gough Physio Rooms Ltd.

We are able to offer you this service at a standard charge. Significant injury risk is possible if you do not follow due diligence and seek suitable professional advice about your injury. No guarantees of specific results are expressly made or implied in this book..